Our Real Health Insurance A-Z And More

Our Real Health Insurance A-Z And More

A Guide For Optimum Wellness And Healing

Dr. Marty Finkelstein

ISBN-13: 9781548141295
ISBN-10: 1548141291
Library of Congress Control Number: 2017909841
CreateSpace Independent Publishing Platform
North Charleston, South Carolina

If you knew the right questions to ask yourself to know about your own health, you'd ask them, wouldn't you? Dr. Finkelstein knows the right questions to ask, and this book is loaded with questions that will help you see through the fog that surrounds health and healing for most people. Dr. Finkelstein has you observe and challenge your beliefs, and through the book helps you to determine how to make better decisions regarding your own health. A must read for anyone desiring greater wellness in their life.
—Dr. Steve Hoffman, author of *Discover Wellness*

Dr. Marty Finkelstein's book takes a holistic look at our current health-care system and educates the reader on the value of integrative therapies and self- care to complement, manage, and insure healthier outcomes. It provides a road map to help us better understand the impact of our choices and what each of us can do to build, nurture, and maintain a healthy mind, body, and spirit from early development through our more seasoned years. It is jam-packed with relatable life stories, experiences, testimonies, personal assessments, examples, and learning tools to help us develop health and wellness strategies we can incorporate on a daily basis to better empower ourselves, our family, friends, and community.
—Belinda Morrow-Stinson-Head, PhD, professional consultant

If you want more energy, less pain, greater flexibility, and more strength, read this book and take control of your own health care. Dr. Finkelstein's strategies are designed to ensure everyday wellness regardless of condition or age.
—Steve Siebold, author of *177 Mental Toughness Secrets of the World Class*

Dr. Finkelstein's new book creates an easy guide for people to discover that their real health insurance is the actions they take in life to improve their physical and emotional well-being. The book is filled with real stories from patients and interactive exercises to engage the reader to look deeper at themselves to achieve optimum wellness.
—Dr. Veronique Desaulniers, author of *Heal Breast Cancer Naturally*

Dr. Marty Finkelstein is a longtime healer in the field of mind body medicine. As Americans, it is time for each of us to take responsibility for staying well. The body holds the wisdom to heal, and this book will put you into alignment with that wisdom.
—Debbie Unterman, master alchemist, author of *Talking to Ourselves*

Once again, Dr. Finkelstein provides us the insight of what it means to be vitally healthy in our body, mind, and spirit. This book is more than just a few tips on how to feel better. It is a guide to creating a way of life for permanent health. While our politicians battle over creating health coverage, we now can create Our Real Health Insurance from A to Z by learning how to get and stay healthy.
—Dr. Joshua Saul, Acupuncturist

Dr. Marty's new book is a wonderful guide for anyone seeking optimum wellness in their life. The interactive stories and exercises engage the reader to realize perhaps becoming healthier does not have to be so complicated. At a time when sickness has become the norm, this book stands as a must read for everyone wanting better health and preventing disease.
—Dr. Michael Norwood, author of *The 9 Insights of the Wealthy Soul*

Once again, we can rely on Dr. Marty Finkelstein to share his wealth of natural healing. As we toll with the variances of health care and health insurance, be assured there is no better insurance than a well-adjusted body that is physically and emotionally motivated, and Dr. Marty is our guide to that end. I highly endorse his efforts and appreciate all he does, as someone who truly cares and shares.
—Dr. Joel Margolies, author of *Smart Start*

The paradigm of healing that Dr. Marty presents in this book explores the *true* meaning of well-being. His insights into the "health care" system are vitally important to understand in today's "crisis care" society. I especially appreciate the important tools and questions that tune the individuals into their internal world (the realm of thoughts and emotions) while interacting in a healthy way with the external world.
—Natalie Rivera, Transformation Services Inc.

Dr. Marty seamlessly blends the physical with the metaphysical, to show how simple actions can have a lasting positive impact on our health. Rather than waiting until disease sets in, make an investment in your health and longevity today! Dr. Marty's multifaceted approach, backed up by his thirty-five years of experience working with patients, teaches us that optimal health comes when we recognize that we are equal parts mind, body, and spirit. After reading *Our Real Health Insurance*, which is filled with wonderful stories and testimonials from patients, I'm inspired to take even greater action to ensure that my health continues to thrive in all areas. Dr. Marty's approach is easy, concise, and easy to understand and follow.
—Meadow Linn, coauthor of *The Mystic Cookbook*

Other books by Dr. Marty Finkelstein

A Life of Wellness, Guidelines for Avoiding Illness

*If Relationships Were Like Sports, Men Would at Least
Know the Score*

*Divorce: An Uncommon Love Story, Healing Your Family, Saving Your Money,
and Renewing Your Life*

The Seven Gifts

8 Lessons of Life on Hole 1

Songs, A Healing Journey

This book is dedicated to all my patients through the years, my friends, and my family, and to each of us who are open to the miracles of life as we open our hearts to continue to discover healing and wellness in our lives.

CONTENTS

PREFACE

HEALTH INSURANCE HAS become more complicated and more expensive than ever before. Even if someone has a great insurance plan with a reasonable premium, there can be high deductibles, copayments, and a percentage that the person may need to pay out of his or her own pocket. Because of the complexity of this problem, there will never be a health plan that is going to make everyone happy. I remember many people I knew were very pleased with Obamacare, yet many people I knew were not happy at all. Some people were able to receive health insurance for the first time, and those with preexisting conditions were also able to receive care without worry that their insurance would be turned down. Some people's premiums went down, while other people's premiums almost doubled. And then there were those who were penalized if they did not participate in the plan. So it is understandable why there are so many mixed emotions regarding health insurance. Should everyone have access to health insurance like they do in many other countries? Or should health insurance not be an entitlement?

This book will not be able to answer all the questions, but it will begin to create a shift in how we think about health insurance to begin with. Most important, it is essential to understand that what has been termed "health insurance" is truly crisis and disease insurance.

I believe everyone should have access to crisis and disease insurance, yet each of us has to learn how to become healthier in our lives to prevent most disease from occurring. These days, if a person is diagnosed with heart disease or diabetes, it is unacceptable if doctors do not spend time explaining the necessity of healthy eating, proper nutrition, and a change of lifestyle. That one shift could save that person's life and save us all the expense of continued disease care and treatment. If each of us were taught the essentials of becoming healthier, by the very health professionals we see, the cost of insurance would be dramatically reduced.

When I was twenty-three years old, I was diagnosed with ulcerative colitis and told there was nothing that could be done to correct this disease other than taking medications, including prednisone, to help control the problem for the rest of my life. I was not explained the consequences of this steroid drug or the devastating side effects it would cause. I was too young and uninformed to even ask appropriate questions. Thankfully, a friend told me about a holistic doctor he was seeing who, through nutrition, chiropractic adjustments, and emotional healing, had corrected his migraine headaches that he had suffered since childhood. I decided to be evaluated by this doctor, and within nine months of following this doctor's treatments and guidance and choosing to not take prednisone and other medications, my ulcerative colitis was improved and ultimately healed. That one decision changed the course of my life, as I learned being healthy is a lifestyle and occurs through understanding "our real health insurance." Simply, information and the choices we make can lead to entirely different outcomes in our lives.

INTRODUCTION

EVERY TIME I give a presentation about health, I ask people in the audience to raise their hand if their health and the health of their family are important to them. Without hesitation, each person raises his or her hand proudly. I then ask those to raise their hand if they can share at least three strategies they have that ultimately create measurable results related to their health and that are part of their lifestyle. Too often the number of hands is few, and all too often the question is asked, "What do you mean by strategies?"

For more than thirty-five years, I have had the blessing of assisting others to greater health and speaking about healing every day. Though sadly, every day I see patients who come to me for the first time and share how they have continued to get sicker and weaker, being diagnosed with various ailments, though it is hardly ever explained how their condition developed and, even more important, how their condition could improve. Interestingly, if we truly began to understand how our health may have declined, it would make even more sense how our health could dramatically change. We just need to know how to change and have specific wellness strategies to measure the results of our improvement.

But there is an inherent problem in our health-care system. At one time medication was specifically used for crisis intervention, after a doctor examined someone, rendered a qualified reason for the medication, and then took the time to explain to their patient what commonsense requirements were necessary to assist the person in regaining his or her health. But today drugs are sold to us, the consumer. The drug companies learned the advertising model from how Coke sells Coke and

McDonald's sells McDonald's. I have patients who empty shopping bags that are filled with their medications in my treatment room just to display all the drugs they take. I wish I can truly say that I have witnessed that the more drugs people take, the healthier they are and become, but instead it is just the opposite. The more drugs we take, the sicker we become, and if we do not identify the true cause of the problem, the more drugs we continue to take, and the more complications regarding our health occur. I know each of you reading this book is indeed interested in becoming healthier, so let me first ask you to answer these simple questions.

1. In your observation as people get older, do they tend to get sicker or healthier?
2. In your observation as people get older, do they tend to need more medication or less?
3. In your observation as people get older, do they need more surgery or less?
4. In your observation as people get older, do they tend to lose function or gain function?
5. Are you getting older?

Considering each of us is indeed getting older, a radical shift of consciousness needs to occur. We need to change the way we take care of ourselves, our approach to our health, and our very core beliefs regarding ourselves and the possibility for ongoing healing in our lives. Drug companies are spending millions of dollars promoting a false concept of wellness, yet they are doing a great job with it, because people are going to their doctors and telling them what drug they want.

We have been led down the road wanting a fast fix to every physical ailment or emotional breakdown that occurs without any regard to consequence. As I flipped through the pages of a popular magazine, I came upon ad after ad promoting medications like candy for a child. One ad spoke of a drug for depression and what wonderful results were manifested after people took this drug. As I scanned down further, in smaller print the ad shared the various side effects that could occur: depression, mood swings, suicidal thoughts, diabetes, anxiety, high blood pressure, and even death. Every day we may read in the paper about the complications of some new drug that had been promoted for pain relief only to find out later of its addictive and devastating qualities.

I believe there is indeed a time for medicine and surgery. As a health-care professional, I refer my patients to other specialists when necessary. Every day, lives are saved with the advancement of technology and the expertise of doctors. I personally have seen the value when all health-care professionals share their unique expertise serving others. On mission trips with Flying Doctors of America, I observed physicians, chiropractors, dentists, therapists, nurses, and volunteers working together to save lives, mend wounds, reduce and prevent infections, help eliminate pain, improve function, and I even witnessed miracles.

On one particular mission trip in Mexico, my health team cared for a young boy with Down syndrome. After I had worked with him for about fifteen minutes, the tension in his body began to ease, his face began to relax, his eyes opened wider, and he began to express a smile. His mother, who was in the room, began to cry, for she had never seen her son smile before that moment. She had believed it was impossible for her little eight-year-old boy to smile.

I believe people need to be reeducated about the wonders and miracles of our own divine power that resides in our body. I believe when people truly understand how healing can occur for each of us at any age and in any condition, they can make clear choices independent of what insurance companies will pay for and honor. Everyone wants to be healthy even when they have been conditioned to believe their illness cannot be helped. All too often one of the most significant side effects of medications taken for years is how they can numb our nervous system, our sense of feeling, and our sense of being connected to the whole person we once were, and sadly disconnect us from our spirit and the very core of our soul and purpose in life. How we respond to ourselves, our friends, and our families can be altered as we become more segmented rather than whole. Even pain is important to listen to, as it speaks through our body like a wise sage trying to get our attention.

I believe we can have a health-care system that is affordable and available to everyone in America, as all health-care professionals work together sharing information and educating our patients. I believe this book can be a guide for each of us to discover "our real insurance" through the choices we make and the actions we take.

Information can lead to inspiration, which can lead to activation, which can lead to transformation.

Part 1
Our Real Health Insurance
A-Z

CHAPTER 1

ATTITUDE/ACTION

ATTITUDE

Our attitude affects our health more than we realize. Though it may sound simplistic, a healthy attitude stimulates healthy cells and a stronger immune system, and an unhealthy attitude can stress our body and lower our resistance to sickness. Attitude, though, is one of those magical things that are hard to define. There is an award-winning documentary called *Happy* that explores the attitudes of people from around the world and why some people who seem to have so little can have a wonderful appreciation for life. We all know when we are around someone who radiates an energy of appreciation. It is easy to be uplifted when around people who are manifesting this quality. Maybe there is an "attitude of appreciation" gene that some people are born with, but I know I have to work my appreciation muscle every day.

"I hear you, Dr. Finkelstein," she said as I quietly walked into her room to give her a treatment. I was treating patients at a nursing home one day a week, and fortunately Anne was one of my patients. She was sitting up, but she no longer had legs and was blind from the long-term effects of diabetes. Yet she always knew when I tiptoed into the room. She was a very beautiful human being. She had the ability to make everyone around her feel better. The nurses, the doctors, and the staff all loved to be in her company because of her amazing attitude. She reminded us all to see what we were blessed with rather than what was missing or challenging in our life. She became my guru, my teacher, for as I worked on her she lifted my spirits.

Once she shared with me about the sadness she felt when her family came to visit her one day with the grandchildren. She often heard the parents reprimanding the children harshly. She told me that though she did not have eyes to see, people with eyes often did not see the harm they did to others by the way they spoke to each other. One day I walked into the room, and she said, "I can see a shadow of you; I am beginning to see." Because of her attitude, she was always open to the possibility of miracles and receiving the healing therapy. She was a gift. A simple person teaching us all lessons to become better in our lives.

QUESTIONS

1. What are four things you appreciate about yourself?
2. What are four things you appreciate about your significant other, child, parent, and sibling?
3. Who do you know in your life who seems to have a great attitude?
4. When is the last time you shared your appreciations with others?
5. When people share something they appreciate about you, how do you feel?
6. Why do you think it sometimes is difficult to share what we appreciate?

Action

We have all heard the expression "actions speak louder than words." As we are understanding our new health insurance, we discover we have to take specific actions to fulfill specific goals. As I earlier mentioned, everyone says that they want to be healthy, yet only about 15 percent of the population actually take the required actions to become healthier. Each goal in life we desire is only realized through the actions that align with those thoughts. Whether it is the actions of exercises, changing eating patterns, choosing to heal from past negative experiences, or seeking guidance, specific results all manifest from the actions we are willing to take. So often people know what they should do to change certain aspects of their life, yet they resist or sabotage taking the necessary actions that are required. So many people in our country alone are overweight and challenged with serious health conditions, and they continue to rationalize not changing the unhealthy habits in their lives. All of us are on the same journey of life together. Our story may be different, but each of us faces challenges and obstacles each day.

Questions

1. What are things you would like to change regarding your physical or emotional health?
2. What actions are you ready to change to manifest those goals?
3. How would you feel about yourself if you were taking those actions?
4. How do you feel when you do not take the actions that you know would lead to reaching your goals? What rational excuses do you say to yourself?

CHAPTER 2

BELIEFS/BREATH OF LIFE

BELIEFS

IF OUR ATTITUDE affects our health, it's our very beliefs that ultimately shape the choices we make in our life and the actions we take. Our life is a mirror of our beliefs. When it comes to our real health insurance, our beliefs hold the answers. The first question we have to ask ourselves is where our beliefs come from. Though we may not think about it, they begin with our parents, and then our upbringing, society, television, radio, the messages we hear all day long, and the things we are taught from a very early age. Sadly, when it comes to our health, most of us have been raised with a belief system that does not support becoming a healthy person. We initially see doctors who prescribe drugs from the earliest age telling parents that these are normal childhood problems that we will simply outgrow without explaining what is truly causing the symptoms. Instead of being outgrown, health conditions become worse. And then we are given more medication, never being informed that there might be alternative approaches that are less harmful and more effective for treating the problems. As we become older, we are led to believe that it's just stress that is affecting our health and told to just continue taking more medication that we are sold each day through television, radio, magazines and the Internet. It is no wonder that by the time we approach forty years old, we have been taught by the same doctors that the degenerative diseases that have occurred over time are simply natural for the aging process. The most degenerative diseases affecting millions of people are heart disease, diabetes, arthritis, and clinical depression.

Imagine if we were taught from early ages that our body could age with vitality and grace if we learned to eat healthy; understood proper exercise; received massage, holistic therapies, and chiropractic care; and learned how to approach emotional challenges in our life in a healthy, healing, transformative way. If we were taught from early childhood how to take care of our body from doctors and parents, just like dentists have taught us how to take care of our teeth, the outcome of our health would be entirely different. I believe most health problems that exist today would be diminished and even eliminated if we truly created beliefs that empowered our life physically, emotionally, and spiritually. In my lifetime there has never been an Olympics where records were not broken. Each Olympics we see striving athletes seeking the best coaches and trainers to enhance peak performance, to simply become better. Imagine if we approached our health with the same attitude and belief. Imagine if we sought out therapists, doctors, and teachers to assist us in becoming our best selves. It is only when we become mindful in our life that we can observe what beliefs we have that diminish our well-being, and what new beliefs we want to create to empower our lives. It is at those moments that our lives can transform.

"I don't believe in chiropractic treatment," she said, as I introduced myself. Glenda was a new patient who shared that she came from a family of medical doctors and worked at the local hospital in the administration department. She said she had been to many orthopedic specialists who were recommending lower-back surgery and that she was in constant pain and had come here as a last hope. After I conducted the examination with Glenda, I shared how I could help her and what would be necessary on her part. I said, "The good news is you don't have to believe in chiropractic care, but you have to be willing to help me help you." She seemed to look a little more relaxed as I shared the treatment schedule and the exercises and therapies that would be required. Then, Glenda shared that she also had suffered from migraine headaches for years and that she was taking ten to fifteen aspirins a day to cope. She said, "If you can also help me with that, it would be a miracle, and I will refer everyone I know to you."

7

One month later Glenda's lower-back pain was 90 percent better, and her headaches were gone. Glenda kept her promise. She referred her children, friends, and members of her church and continued to get better.

Sometimes our beliefs are manifested by the commitments and actions we choose.

Questions

1. What are your beliefs about your health?
2. Can you see how your beliefs affect the actions you take regarding your own health, and ultimately your life?
3. If you were taught to take a drug for every symptom and never taught to understand what was causing that symptom, can you see how that would affect the actions you took and the outcome of your health?
4. Do you believe you can change unhealthy habits like smoking, poor nutrition, lack of exercise, and negative emotional patterns in your life?

Breath of Life

Yes, breathing is the most essential component of life and being alive. If I could show someone only one exercise, it would be the art of learning to mindfully breathe deeply. Sadly, as people become older and are doing less aerobic activity, they are getting less than the necessary amount of oxygen for each of the billions of cells in our body to generate new, healthy cells. When we are children, we tend to be active by the very nature of playing and participating in sports and activities. Yet even now children are less active and becoming more sedentary with computers, games, and texting.

What we call our normal breathing pattern is an automatic shallow breath, just enough to survive but not enough to assist the body in regenerating and becoming healthier. We have to learn to consciously breathe deeper through simple exercises and strategies during the day. We have to make the time to pause during the day and remind ourselves to breathe in through our nose for the count of five, hold it in for the count of five, breathe out for the count of five, and then hold it out for the count of five, and repeat this cycle for thirty seconds a few times a day. Learning to breathe deeply immediately reduces stress in the body and can lower blood pressure, relax muscles, and get more oxygen to the brain and other organs to function healthier. Breathing deeply and slowly is important to our health and vitality because it immediately changes the physical and emotional physiology of the body. Often women who are pregnant will participate in birthing classes where they are taught the importance of breathing deeply when they feel pain. Unknowingly, our immediate reaction to pain is holding our breath and tightening our muscles. This is a survival instinct of the body going into a protective or guarded reflex. But the outcome actually causes more complications, as the blood flow and oxygen intake into the muscles becomes restricted. The goal is breathing deeper to get more oxygen into the blood, bringing nutrients to muscles that help the muscles relax.

Just the other day, a patient, Ms. Hartford, came into the office and shared that she had to go see the emergency nurse at work because she felt anxious and nauseous. When they took her blood pressure, it was 205/115. This is extremely high and dangerous. They recommended she start taking blood-pressure medication, which she was reluctant to do. I explained to her how and why blood pressure can elevate in the body and why sometimes medication, though not the solution, can be necessary. I proceeded to give her an adjustment through a technique called B.E.S.T. This stands for bio energetic synchronization technique which is a non–forceful energy balancing procedure to reestablish the full healing potential of the body.

During the treatment I coached her in breathing slowly and deeply, which at first was very difficult for her. After ten minutes I could feel her body relaxing, as her breathing pattern became easy and effortless. I could feel her muscles beginning to relax, as a wave of peacefulness began to glow from her face. After the adjustment I took her blood pressure, and it was 123/84, which is a healthy blood-pressure reading. I explained to her that it was going to be necessary to follow up on her blood-pressure readings each day and monitor her overall health. I shared with her the importance of following the guidelines to become healthier and at the same time being evaluated by her medical doctor with a clearer understanding of her own health. But what would have occurred if someone did not have any other treatment alternatives? The person would have begun taking the blood-pressure medication without understanding what was causing the problem. Most medical doctors are taught to respond efficiently to the crisis with drug intervention without explaining in detail what is essentially causing the crisis and how to truly become healthier.

I recommend that each day we begin to take two to three deep breaths throughout the day. The next time you are sitting in traffic, waiting on line in the grocery store, working at your job, watching television, or engaged on your computer, simply pause, take thirty seconds, and breathe. There is a reason it is called the Breath of Life.

Breathing Exercise Review

If you have difficulty breathing in through your nose, begin by first blowing out your mouth as if you were blowing out five birthday candles. Allow yourself to exhale all the way until you feel your abdominal muscles tighten. Count to five before you breathe in through your nose as if you were inhaling the fragrance of a divine healing flower. Breathe in for the count of five. Then hold it in for five seconds before you blow out your mouth again. The more you practice the Breath of Life, the easier it will become, and the more health benefits you will experience. Begin doing this every day throughout the day for thirty seconds.

CHAPTER 3

CONSISTENCY/COMMITMENT/CHANGE

YOU CAN BEGIN to see that each of these strategies for your real health insurance begin to connect with each other. It is very much like learning to cultivate a garden and discovering how each aspect becomes an essential part of the whole. One strategy in itself will not achieve the desired results. It is the alchemy of all the ingredients coming together. Like in the garden, water is essential, but without soil, without nutrients, without consistency, without sunshine, and without cultivation, the garden will on its own simply become a garden of sickly weeds.

One of the greatest challenges we all seem to face is the commitment to change unhealthy habits into healthy habits. How often have we heard someone else say, "I have always been this way; it's just the way I am"? Well, one of the greatest gifts we have is our ability to change. In truth it is one of the major distinctions that separate us from being like another highly trained mammal. Imagine if your very smart dog today decided to be a vegetarian for a week as an experiment. As smart as your dog might be, his cerebral cortex does not have the capability to make that decision. Thankfully we do. Yet too often we do not exercise that ability that we possess. We often say, "It is so hard to change," but we can change!

All of us can be inspired to change especially when we want the desired outcome. Most of us learned to ride a bicycle and drive a car, even though both activities were extremely challenging. Remember how often you fell learning to ride that bike? Yet you continued to get back on, because your desire was greater than all the reasons you had to quit. It took time; it took consistency and commitment; yet you succeeded.

And it was a great feeling when you did. When we make commitments and we are consistent in our actions, we ultimately nurture our own spirit and feel better about ourselves. This has become more difficult in our culture, because we are all looking for fast solutions to every challenge in our life. We are told we need medication to feel better but not told what we need to do to become healthier. We see so many quick fixes to lose weight, and so many diets that often people begin a diet and then predictably stop shortly after. We are told we can achieve success without even working. All of us would like to believe that with a few piano lessons, we could play like Mozart, or that we could become a great athlete in thirty days or become healthy by taking this one herb. It would be wonderful if it were true. But it is not! Our real health insurance requires commitment and the consistency of learning new information, being inspired, and taking action to discover how our health and life can transform.

Marge was a thirty-six-year-old woman assisted into the office by her husband. She needed a cane to support herself. She explained that she was diagnosed with multiple sclerosis and that the doctors shared that she would probably need a wheelchair within nine months. A good friend of hers had recommended she come see me for an evaluation. After a thorough examination and consultation, it was clear that she was not eating healthy, nor did she have any exercise protocol. She was still young and thin and was very weak and frail. I told her that I did not know how much I could help her, considering the circumstances and complications of multiple sclerosis. I recommended that she follow my treatment plan for about six months, which included following my nutritional guidelines, and begin doing the exercises I demonstrated for her each day. I said that if we observed her body getting stronger and improving, then we would both decide what course of action to continue to take. I told her that this was going to take a commitment on her part and the willingness to change and be consistent in her actions for me to help her. Well, within six months she was back working and walking without any cane, and she continued to follow many of my recommendations through the next twenty-nine years. Her multiple-sclerosis doctors did not understand how she continued to improve, but sadly they never called me to find out what procedures, therapies, and treatments I have used to assist her to greater health.

Questions

1. What changes have you made regarding your health in the last five years?
2. What are changes you would like to make regarding your health?
3. How do you feel about yourself when you keep your commitments?
4. How do you feel about yourself when you break your commitments?
5. What is one thing you are ready to change to improve your health starting today?

CHAPTER 4

DARE TO DREAM

ONE OF THE healthiest qualities a child can develop is the capacity to dream. It is through our aspirations and dreams that we naturally evolve, fulfilling on actions in our life that bring out the best in us. We are all familiar with Martin Luther King's "I have a dream" speech. Each of us has dreams and desires that motivate us in our lives even through some of the greatest challenges. You may have a dream to become successful, to achieve fame, to become a great athlete, to have a wonderful family, to see your children develop into healthy adults pursuing their own dreams, to be the best person you can be, to travel the world, or to simply find joy and happiness in the simple pleasures of life. Our dreams awake us in the morning with excitement, greeting the day with powerful visions and affirmations. When we are young, dreaming is as natural as walking. Children allow their imagination to play with possibilities. I can remember when I was around ten years old my teachers labeling me as a dreamer in school. I wish I could have had teachers who inspired my dreams. But as we get older, our dreams can begin to diminish. Perhaps we have accomplished many of our dreams or seen our dreams not be fully realized, leaving us frustrated. But it is indeed the dream of tomorrow that excites the actions of today. As we age and begin looking at our time of retirement, it is essential to discover new dreams that bring excitement to our lives. As I am approaching those ages, I am facing this myself as I search for my purpose in the next phase of life. The purpose of dreaming is not necessarily to change the world but to change the world that you are living in. It takes courage to dream, to be the best you can be.

Thirty years ago, Steve, a young twenty-three-year-old who had played championship junior tennis, became my friend and patient. He shared with me his dreams of becoming very successful in his life. Steve had a strong desire to feel his best physically, emotionally, and nutritionally. His excitement fused with his dreams was contagious. He was willing to change old patterns that did not support his goals, and he was willing to create new patterns to achieve his dreams. It was a joy assisting him toward manifesting his life's true purpose.

Well, he has fulfilled his dreams and continues to do so. He is one of the leading experts in achieving success and wealth in life, and he continues traveling the world sharing his expertise with thousands of people. One must dream big to achieve lofty goals!

Questions

1. If you are single, what would a dream date be for you?
2. If you are in a relationship, what would a dream vacation be for you?
3. If you were physically able to accomplish anything, what would you like to do?
4. What would a dream job look like for you?
5. What is your dream home?
6. If you inherited one million dollars, what would you do with it?
7. What is your dream for our planet and all the people in it?

Have fun playing with your dreams.

CHAPTER 5

EXERCISE/EMOTIONS

EXERCISE

THERE ARE HUNDREDS of books about the benefits of exercise, as well as the various types of exercise. I think everyone knows that exercise plays a vital role regarding our health and wellness. Yet I still see so many people confused and frustrated when it comes to integrating exercise in their lifestyle. All too often we slip into that immediate-result mind-set and begin an exercise program that our body is not ready for, and we sadly injure our muscles or joints. Exercise, like every other strategy for becoming healthier, needs specific goals, applications, and accountability. I can understand why so many people are confused and frustrated, though, because many of the experts say that we need to exercise for about an hour five days a week to receive the benefits for our cardiovascular conditioning. Most of us live in front of computers and television screens, on our smartphones, and in our cars commuting each day. None of this counts as healthy exercise for our bodies. But most people are simply not going to be able to find an hour four to five days a week and continue it for a lifestyle. For those people who are making the time and enjoying the results of their commitment, continue to do so. But most of us get inspired by the commercials selling exercise equipment and the ads that promote quick results, and we believe the hype without understanding the journey.

Exercise is like building a house, and it all depends on where your house is beginning. For some it starts with a blueprint, someone to help you design a vision for what you want to create. For some there is already a strong foundation to build upon. For some the house has been there, but it's remodeling time, time to get excited again, and change things around with a new perspective. For some it is developing a bigger house with a whole new blueprint to create a bigger vision. If someone has not had any healthy habit of exercise, it should begin with simple daily exercises that take just a few minutes each day at home. I am a believer in everyday simple exercises wherever we are. Regardless of your strategy, it is essential to have everyday stretching and strengthening routines, even if they are only five minutes a day.

Imagine if every day you were stretching starting when you were young and knew how far you could stretch. Imagine if every day you consciously observed how your body felt when you stretched, what was tight or sore, and what felt better or worse, consistently twice a day. Imagine if every day you did twenty push-ups twice a day, observing your body, starting when you were young. Imagine if every day you jumped rope for thirty seconds twice a day, observing your stamina and endurance. So if you could imagine this, the question is at what age would you not be able to do these things? Would you one day bend half as far, not be able to jump rope, only be able to do three push-ups? The obvious answer is you would be able to do all these things and continue to be able to do these things, aging with grace and vitality, especially if you were applying all the strategies of becoming healthier in your life.

One of the most important keys to exercise is learning to breathe correctly. We already shared about the essence of breathing, so now you can understand its importance even deeper. For any exercise we do, breathing correctly will add to the results of that exercise 95 percent. If you do not learn how to breathe properly, you will diminish your overall strength, endurance, and capacity to improve.

I was once working on an Olympic marathon runner. I watched Sally run and gave her my feedback, which she desired, because she was committed to improving her overall time and ability to improve and reduce injuries. I explained three things that would accomplish her goals. One was getting a few chiropractic adjustments to reduce the tightness in her upper back, neck, and lower back while aligning her spine and nervous system. Two was focusing on relaxing her neck, shoulders, and arms when she ran. And the other was breathing slowly, in through her nose and out through her mouth in a steady rhythm. The next time I saw her to give her an adjustment, she excitedly shared how she had applied those things I recommended and had broken her own best time in a marathon. The beauty of healthy strategies, whether it is for athletes striving to be their best or a person wanting to become healthier, is that we soon discover that improvement is measureable and predictable. Regardless of the stage you are in designing your exercise home, these are strategies I recommend for everyone regardless of age or condition to be able to do at home or anywhere.

EXERCISE STRATEGIES

1. Comfort-zone stretching: Every morning and evening when you first wake up and before you go to sleep, gently stretch your legs and back within your comfort-zone limitations. This means that if you have a problem, do not aggravate that muscle or joint, but discover what stretch you can do painlessly. Comfort-zone stretching can be simple yoga exercises or gentle bending and turning.

2. Breathing in through your nose and gently out through your mouth while stretching. If you have ever done yoga, take a few simple exercises you have learned and apply them each day in your life.

3. Magic jump rope: This is not for everyone but for those who can comfortably jump. The magic jump rope is your personal invisible jump rope to use twice a day for thirty seconds. No more tripping or clunking yourself in the arms or shoulders, but truly imagine using your arms and legs, while breathing in the proper rhythm.

4. Stretchy bands: These are inexpensive elastic bands that can be purchased at Target. These bands are great for strengthening

muscles and stretching areas of your body. I take a band with me wherever I go. Of course, with any exercise it is essential that you consult with a specialist to show you how to exercise the best way, so that you are not injuring yourself. I teach people how to do ten exercises with one stretchy band.

5. Tai chi modifications: Tai chi is a part of martial arts using slow movement with breathing to balance the nervous system. It is great to learn tai chi as well as chi gong. But what I recommend to people who enjoy playing tennis or golf is to apply the principles of these techniques each day, practicing their swings in slow motion and feeling the movement of their body. When you do go on the tennis court or golf course, these muscles will already have a muscle memory, allowing your swing to feel more at ease, which will also help avoid injuries.

6. If you like to dance, have fun dancing to music at home.

7. Modified sit-ups and push-ups. This can be push-ups against a wall, and sit-ups where you gently bend forward without straining.

Make exercise fun!

EMOTIONS

In this book is a section specifically on emotional healing because of the significance it can have regarding our overall healing and health. I believe how we respond to stress in our lives affects our health more than we realize. Every day we hear how stressed people are in their lives. But sadly, we have made stress a cliché rather than truly understanding the underlying cause of the stress in our lives. Stress can have physical, nutritional, chemical, or many times emotional factors that are causing physiological reactions in the body. Too often we do not realize we literally bring our stress with us wherever we go. In other words the stress many times is not because of the external factors, but more related to the internal factors—the very conversations we are having with ourselves.

One day I had a patient come into the office sharing how upset he was that he had just lost his job. His body was tense, his blood pressure was higher than usual, and it was even difficult for him to breathe. A few hours later, another patient came in who immediately started venting about the stress in his day. He looked like he was about to have a heart attack right there in my office. I asked what had happened. He mentioned that he was building his million-dollar dream home on the lake and could not get his builders and contractors to show up on time. I told him, "Well, let's give you a great treatment so you can at least feel relaxed and embrace the blessings of your success." A few patients later, another patient came in. She shared she had just lost her job because the company she was working for was downsizing. I said that I was sorry to hear that, to which she replied, "Don't be; it's the best thing to happen." She told me that she had been working there nine years and not fulfilling her real desires and passions. She was excited about now having the time to start her own business, which was always her dream.

One of the strategies of becoming healthier is becoming conscious of our thoughts and emotions. Most of us are moving so fast we do not even realize the thoughts and emotions that are pulling our strings from inside us. Every relationship we are in is directly affected by our ability to communicate effectively and honestly about our thoughts and feelings.

In our society we have been taught to stuff feelings in, to not feel what we are feeling, to intellectualize what we are feeling rather than create the space to feel what we feel. There is a saying, "Feeling is healing." We have so many people who are put on medications to not feel the emotional challenges in their lives. When this occurs human beings do not develop an emotional IQ. Challenges are normal in life, as is stress, and the very essence of learning to become healthier enables us to respond to these challenges in healthier ways. This ultimately causes our immune and nervous systems to become more efficient and more sophisticated. As we approach health with healthy strategies, we need less medication, and we begin looking at the true cause of our body's symptoms.

Dorothy came in the next day after her initial treatment. She shared how relaxed she was after her healing session. She mentioned that night she went home and had the most peaceful sleep. When she awoke, she had a revelation. She realized that it was the first time since she was a child that she had slept with the light off. She never could explain to her husband or anyone why she felt she needed the light on during the night. But then it became clear that some experience had been pushed deep within her all these years that affected her trust, her sharing, and her overall vitality in every relationship she was in, including the most important relationship, the one with herself. She remembered that she was sexually abused as a little girl, and there was no one to ever talk about it with her. She looked at me with tears in her eyes and shared that she felt at peace and free for the first time in her life. She felt she no longer needed to hold on to those memories and this pain. And she understood for the first time why she had felt so much fear in her life that seemed to affect everything.

In my book *Divorce: An Uncommon Love Story*, I share my own turbulent emotional challenges through my own divorce. It was a time when moments of rage, anger, sadness, and grief were all present. Thankfully, applying everything I knew, I began a journey to facilitate healing for myself as well as my family. During those difficult times, I developed deeper compassion, understanding, forgiveness, and love, which allowed a transformation to evolve in my family. My greatest fear was that my children would be raised in a typical divorce, where the anger of both parents affected our children, making their life more difficult. Instead, the outcome was my children experiencing their parents becoming best friends and wonderful parenting partners. It was only through understanding true healing that this very challenging time in my life became a time of deep evolving and transformation.

Questions

1. Are there areas in your past relationships that feel unresolved?
2. What are your emotional challenges you feel with your family?
3. What are the emotional challenges you feel at work?
4. What actions in your life have you taken or want to take to become healthier in those areas?

CHAPTER 6

FAITH/FUN/FORGIVENESS

FAITH

HAVING FAITH IS an essence of believing. Our real health insurance is an alchemy of many ingredients, and faith is an essential one. Having faith is a manifestation of many actions we take in life. We all can develop a deeper faith when we achieve our goals through vision and commitment. Our faith is a seed that needs to be nurtured and tended to just like the seeds of a garden. Faith is developing a spirit that envisions what we desire while our actions align with those goals and dreams. If you desire to lose weight or lower your blood pressure, it is mandatory that your actions are those that can reach those goals. But faith is necessary to pull us forward even when the road is difficult and distractions occur. Faith is a process of surrendering. All we ultimately can do is be our best, do our best, keep our integrity, and then let go of what we cannot control or even understand at the time. If you are planting a garden, you learn all the things you need to do to have a healthy garden. And then you have faith in the very process of life itself. From that magical seed can develop the miracle of a beautiful tomato. Who truly understands the chemistry, physics, biology, and quantum physics of how life itself works? Yet we know that miracles of life can manifest when we are diligent in our deeds. Our very health is no different from that tomato seed. We are all composed of trillions of cells that require tending to, nurturing our physical, nutritional, and emotional healing. Miracles can occur when we align our faith with our actions each day.

They brought him into the room to be worked on. They said his name was Anthony. His body was trembling from his head down to his feet. I was on a medical mission trip in the Dominican Republic. He lay on the table as I began to work on him. I was told that he had fallen into an open pit fire when he was a little boy, and ever since then he had these continuous, involuntary tremors. They told me through the interpreters that he came here "in faith" to be healed. After about twenty minutes, his body began to relax, and the trembling began to diminish. As he relaxed deeper, I could feel the subtle energies of his body begin to align and balance. The muscles around his face began to relax as he gently exposed a smile, letting go of any fear that had been imbedded into the memory of his body. When I had him come off the table, he stood calm and peaceful. I asked the interpreters to tell him that he no longer had anything to be afraid of. When they shared this with him, tears instantly broke from his eyes, and he embraced me. At that moment he reclaimed his freedom from an incident that had occurred when he was a child and that had caused physical pain and emotional fear. I was witness to the miracle as much as anyone else there. But it was his faith that morning that had him walk miles to our mission site and surrender to the possibility of healing.

Faith always aligns with specific actions.
Faith without action is wishing.

FUN

What do you do for fun? Life can become filled with the stress of duties, responsibilities, and challenges relating to finances, health, work, and relationships. It is essential for the healthy spirit to discover things you enjoy and make the time to have fun doing them. We often hear people say that certain activities reduce stress in their lives. Scientists have discovered healthy cells are produced when people are having fun. The secret is to find your fun and have fun in what you do. Sometimes I hear many of my patients say they just don't have time. They are tired from their long day at work or their work at home. It becomes easy to simply become resigned, doing little to change any habits. Sadly, they become more stressed and eventually depressed. I have seen so many of my patients transform their lives once they are willing to make the time to discover a fun activity.

FUN ACTIVITIES

1. Write down five fun activities. It could be anything—painting, biking, cooking, dancing, singing, traveling, playing an instrument, playing a sport, or going on a nature walk. Think about what might be fun for you.
2. How do you think you would feel after taking the time to have some fun?
3. When was the last thing you did that was fun?
4. What is a fun activity you have always wanted to do?
5. What reasons do you tell yourself for not taking the time to do something that would be fun?
6. What were fun things you did as a child?
7. If you are in an intimate relationship, what do you both do to have fun?
8. When the relationship first began, what did you both do to have fun?

Forgiveness

In all spiritual teachings, there is the consistent message of forgiveness. Forgiveness is more powerful than any drug we can take, and instead of numbing and suppressing our emotional pain, we discover the healing process of the human spirit. It is a difficult journey for anyone to learn how to forgive when the horrors of pain dig so deep. All of us have been hurt to some degree, yet with many the atrocities are difficult to even imagine. Yet it is only in forgiveness that we ourselves become free from the anger, the hate, the shame, the rage, the judgments, and the revenge. But how do we learn to forgive? I have found it worthy to study the lives of people whose very life radiates the spirit of forgiveness. If we read about the lives of Nelson Mandala, Desmond Tutu, the Dali Lama, Martin Luther King Jr., Buddha, Gandhi, and Jesus, we can discover the deep-rooted spiritual understanding and importance of forgiveness. All of us have the capacity to forgive, but it is a muscle that requires tending to like any muscle, and most important, we must learn to forgive ourselves.

As we begin to develop the heart of forgiveness, we bring that gift for others to see what is possible in their own lives. The words "Forgive them; they know not what they do," echoed by Jesus, are words that convey deep understanding into the nature of humankind and the wisdom of spiritual forgiveness. As we learn to forgive, we develop a deeper love, compassion, and wisdom in this journey of life. Forgiveness frees us from the disease of toxic emotions that can aggravate our vitality and health. Yet learning to forgive, truly forgive, can take time. As we continue to heal ourselves, forgiveness becomes inevitable.

During my own separation and divorce, I was filled with anger and rage. On one very specific occasion, I spontaneously prayed and asked for guidance during this challenging moment. I could feel the horror of my life spinning out of control and becoming a person I did not want to be. How would I live with myself, I thought, if nothing changed? Within a few minutes of being in a meditative prayer, I heard a voice speak to me that said, "In your darkest rage and anger, you will discover even deeper love, compassion, and forgiveness." When I came out from my meditation, I felt a new peacefulness as rage and anger was released, and most important, I saw a new vision for my family where healing could be possible for all of us. That moment transformed my life, and the power of forgiveness was actualized. That moment has stayed within my spirit ever since. That voice with those words has continued to be a mantra in my life every day.

Forgiveness in Your Life

1. Who in your life do you still feel resentment or anger toward?
2. What do you judge yourself about?
3. Do you believe you have healthy relationships with each person in your family? Is there healthy communication?
4. Imagine if you felt free from the judgments, the blame, and the anger. Imagine if you felt no you longer had to prove anything to anyone or be defensive about anything. Imagine how you would feel if you felt true forgiveness in your heart.

CHAPTER 7

GRATEFUL

EACH DAY COMES with opportunities and challenges. Yet in the midst of the external forces of life, we can be reminded of the blessings and things to be grateful for. As simple as this may seem, it tends to be difficult for most of us to verbalize to ourselves and others. Every day healing should consist of a grateful exercise. I have found this exercise difficult when I am feeling stressed and even can sense my resistance when my energy is out of balance. Yet the moment I begin sharing what I am grateful for, I can immediately feel a shift in my body and spirit taking place. If you are in an intimate relationship, a wonderful exercise is to share with each other what you feel grateful for about yourself and then about the other person. But don't stop there; this exercise can be implemented into each relationship you are in to bring deeper compassion, trust, appreciation, respect, and love. Gratefulness is the food that nurtures the spirit and expands our consciousness, which in essence attracts to us more abundance to be grateful for. So often in life, we are so busy trying to achieve more that we forget to take the time to pause and be grateful for what we have.

Carla was eighty two years old with blue eyes the color of the sky and hair silver white the color of the clouds when she first came to my office. She told me that she had been a portrait painter her whole life and taught portrait painting up till five years ago. She hated giving up painting. It was her love, but she no longer felt she had the physical or mental strength to continue. Carla told me she did not like taking medication but had developed a severe infection that had caused her leg to swell making it difficult to walk. She had seen her medical doctor and had been taking prednisone, but did not want to continue taking the medicine.

I told Carla that problems like she was having could be aggravated by refined food particularly those loaded with sugar. Her eyes opened wide as she confessed that she loved to eat sweets. I asked her if she would be willing to give up sweets while I adjusted and balanced her nervous system over the next month. There was a slight hesitation, and then she said she was ready.

By the end of that month the swelling in her leg had gone down about ninety percent. On her next visit she shared how grateful she was for all of my help. And then she said that since receiving these treatments she had been feeling more energy and deeper concentration and wanted to start painting again. And the first portrait painting she wanted to do; was me.

That painting hangs in my office with Carla's story written out next to it sharing how grateful she was to be doing what she loves doing once again.

QUESTIONS

1. What are three things you are grateful for in your life?
2. If you are in an intimate relationship, what are three things you are grateful for regarding your partner?
3. If you have children, what are three things you are grateful for regarding each one of them?
4. What are you grateful for regarding your career path?

CHAPTER 8

HUMOR/HOLISTIC HEALING

HUMOR

NORMAN COUSINS, A physician, wrote a book years ago called *Anatomy of an Illness*. Dr. Cousins had been diagnosed with a severe life-threatening degenerative disease and told by the other medical experts that he probably had little time left here on Earth. He decided that instead of taking all the pain medication and staying in the hospital, he would enjoy the time he had left. One of the things he decided was to begin to watch the movies that had made him laugh the most when he was a younger man and child. Interestingly, he discovered that the more he laughed, the better he felt, and his pain began to diminish. As time went on, it was discovered that his disease went into remission. It was as if the laughter created healthy, strong, happy cells in his body, defeating the disease cells. Dr. Cousins went on to write that book and many others, touring the world for many years as one of the most sought-out speakers in the wellness and holistic field. He became an advocate of healthy foods, specific supplements, and holistic body work to assist the body and mind in becoming healthier. Instead of dying in a few months, Dr. Cousins lived several years before he did eventually make his transition. He left with us all a story of hope, the willingness to change, inspiration, and the importance of laughter and humor in our lives. We all love to be around people who make us laugh. Women often say that being with someone with a good sense of humor who can make them laugh is essential for an intimate relationship.

Jean, who has been one of my patients over the years, has a very infectious laugh. When Jean comes in for her monthly adjustments, we always share a few stories that tend to initiate her delightful laughter. The sound of her laughter is heard throughout the whole office. When I enter the room with the next patient, they always request to have the same adjustment that Jean received.

Questions

1. What are three movies or television shows that make you laugh?
2. What comedians do you think are funny?
3. Do you think you are funny or humorous at times?
4. Which of your friends or family members can make you laugh?

HOLISTIC HEALING

This whole book shares insights, information, and stories regarding holistic healing. When we observe the body, mind, and spirit holistically or as a whole interconnected, we begin to easily perceive the importance of healthy strategies in our lives. Most of us have been raised in an allopathic model of medicine. That means we see a different doctor for each different part of the body. We have medical doctors who specialize, treating the body all too often as if the parts are not connected to the whole. We may see a heart specialist for the heart, who may refer us to an orthopedic doctor for our bones, then to an allergy specialist, who might make a referral to a gastrointestinal doctor. So often patients are seeing several different doctors who are prescribing different medications to treat the conditions they are specializing in, while the patient is having various side effects from the multitude of the medication. It starts when we are children, taking medication for symptoms but not necessarily correcting the underlying cause of the condition. A holistic approach to health begins to ask what might be causing the symptoms or illness from a physical, nutritional, or emotional perspective. In many cases all three are involved.

Our Real Health Insurance does not diminish the need for medication, medical evaluations, or surgery when it is necessary, but it suggests that the ongoing lifetime measures of taking medication or removing organs or tissues from the body ultimately never addresses the cause of the health problems or assists the body in becoming healthier. A simple example might be someone who lives through a heart attack and thankfully is saved through emergency surgery. This person is placed on medication that will be required for the rest of his or her life. I have had hundreds of patients come into my office after serious emergency situations like this, yet they have never been informed what caused their heart attack and what healthy strategies need to occur to assist in preventing further complications to their health. If these people do not change their nutritional, physical, and emotional patterns in their lifestyle, they will continue to have further degenerative conditions developing, as well as serious consequences and side effects from the ongoing increase of medication that will be necessary. This will mean very expensive procedures in hospitals and further surgeries and tests on a continuing basis. The problem remains that health-insurance costs escalate, but people do not get healthier unless we change our approach to our health and health concerns. If each of us started when we were children to be taught about having a healthy body, just like we are educated to have healthy teeth, then being and becoming healthier would be a normal and natural journey of life. Eating healthy and simple exercise every day would be strategies that we truly looked forward to.

The Holistic Model of Health

PHYSICAL

1. What do you do to improve your physical well-being? How often do you exercise? What physical activities are you engaged in?

NUTRITIONAL

2. Do you eat healthy every day? What are the foods you know you should begin eliminating from your diet? Do you feel you understand what healthy foods you should be eating each day?

EMOTIONAL/MENTAL

3. What are you doing to improve your emotional development to create healthier relationships?
4. How would you say you respond to stress in your life? Do you feel you can have a healthy, loving conversation with the people you care about in your life? What have you learned about yourself from past and present relationships?

CHAPTER 9

INFORMATION/INSPIRATION

INFORMATION

THIS BOOK IS all about information so that all of us can make wise choices regarding our true health insurance. Information is the basic ingredient where wellness begins. Thankfully, we live in a time where information is more available than ever before. Any person can access the Internet, watch informative shows on television, and gather information that could change the person's life for the better. Too often we do not realize how information has affected the way we think about our health in an adverse way. We have been raised on commercials selling us processed junk food and fast food that is loaded with salt, unhealthy fats, sugars, additives, harmful chemicals, and artificial flavors and colors, and then raised on commercials selling us drugs to mask symptoms as a life choice. So the true question is what information do we have, and where is that information coming from, and does the information empower or diminish our health?

Of course, the information in itself is not responsible for our actions, but it is a powerful fuel for how we think. When the fast-food industry considered selling less processed food, they decided they were in the business of making money, and people could decide for themselves what they wanted to eat. At that moment they all agreed to increase the amount of money they spent selling us their artificial, unhealthy foods. When I first opened my office in 1982, there were no mega bookstores, there were no computers, and there were just a few health-food stores. When people first came to see me, there was limited information available for them to read unless they were already a student of holistic wellness. Now we live in an abundant information age. A true miracle can occur when we receive information that can transform our health and it inspires us to take healthy action.

When Pecolia was first a patient of mine, I could tell she was digesting all the information I was sharing with her. Though she was already in her sixties, her eyes were lighting up like a child in a toy store. She had never had a doctor explain how the body worked before and how our health could improve. She would also purchase the books I had already written about physical health and emotional healing, and pretty soon she was coming for her visit and requesting ten books she could share with friends and family. One day the person who was working for me did not show up, and Pecolia after her treatment asked if I needed any assistance. "Well, if you simply answer the phone, that would be great," I replied. Shortly after that, Pecolia left her job and began working in my office, simply because she wanted to be around the environment of healing and wellness. Soon after, she was the office manager, a devoted friend, and someone whom I truly appreciated, respected, and admired. I believe information is a bridge that can change us and change the world.

QUESTIONS

1. What books have you read that have inspired you in your life?
2. Do you ever search for information on the Internet to learn more?
3. Do you ever watch videos to learn more about a specific subject?
4. Where have you received your information regarding health?

Inspiration

Everyone knows eating healthy has tremendous benefits for our health. Everyone knows that the proper exercise can improve our vitality, strength, and wellness. Yet the problem is approximately 85 percent of the population does not take the action to change habits in their life. Information is the first ingredient for change, but inspiration is the fire, the energy that motivates us to succeed. Unless we are inspired, we will remain unmotivated and lazy when it comes to the most important aspects of our life. Inspiration that leads to action to fulfill goals and visions ultimately has us feel better about ourselves. When we make commitments toward better health, we feel better physically, emotionally, and spiritually. We become more positive in our life and reconnect to our true source of inner confidence and willpower. We begin to believe in ourselves.

As you can see, our real health insurance is a process of many thoughts and actions that are all interconnected with each other. Little changes lead to more changes and lead to reaching our desires and goals. Inspiration, though, is a muscle that needs to be exercised each day. Like a fire the flame will quickly diminish if one is not adding the essentials it needs. All of us can get into lazy patterns, feel depressed, feel the challenges in life that weigh us down, be told that nothing can be done and that we're getting too old, and feel like we have tried in the past and only failed. Each of us has the possibility to become healthier regardless of condition or age if we are willing to hear new information, or old information with new ears and a new brain, and be inspired to make passionate commitments.

In the last thirty-five years, patients have heard me explain about the body in ways they never understood before. Things that should have been explained starting when they were young. Often I see people become excited and inspired as they discover that they can begin to feel better, have more energy, be able to do more, and prevent future problems while needing less medication and surgery. Medication will not give us inspiration. Many times the more medication we take, the more we begin to lose the desire to change. We lose the feelings of being inspired, and we simply continue taking more medication, hoping that our health will improve. But instead problems become more complicated, leading to further illness. The cycle of disease continues as we become sicker, having less energy and feeling less inspired. In that sickness model, we simply continue adapting to illness as a perfectly normal phase of life. But it isn't! Inspiration comes from the word *inspire*. To breathe in the breath of life, we reawaken ourselves to become inspired once again in our lives. Inspiration is deeply connected to our spiritual creative force. When we feel creative in our life, we are igniting the fires of inspiration. All of us are creative beings. Some of us have been inspired by others to pursue our creative dreams, while others have been sedated to the point of diminishing our creative inspirational energies. Inspiration is a power that with focus, action, and vision can achieve many of the goals in our life.

Mr. Peterson was brought into my office by a very good patient of mine. She had asked me if I treated patients in wheelchairs, which I did. When I met Mr. Peterson, I learned that he was born with cerebral palsy yet managed to obtain a degree from college, had become a minister, was an author of his autobiography, hosted a television show, and had met personally with Jimmy Carter. He was now a man in his fifties, and even though his speech was slow, his wisdom and healing spirit lit up the office. When I asked my patient why Mr. Peterson was here to see me, she replied that she had told him about my office and about my holistic chiropractic approach to health, and he said he wanted to see me and to be worked on to feel better. Every time Mr. Peterson enters my office, he inspires me to become the best I can be!

QUESTIONS

1. Can you remember a time you felt inspired?
2. How do you attempt to inspire others in your life?

3. Do you remember a time someone seemed to put out your inspirational fire?
4. When you feel your creative, inspired force, how do you feel about life and yourself?
5. Are there people in your life you share your inspirations with? Do you feel empowered or judged?

As I breathe in today, I feel inspired in my life.

CHAPTER 10

JOY

WHAT BRINGS JOY to your life? Do you know that joy creates endorphins in our body that are relaxing and healing? Joy comes in various shapes and sizes for people. Some people have a wonderful sense of joy cultivating their garden, others cooking and preparing wonderful, creative meals. Joy can occur from serving others, even volunteering one's time to organizations that one feels strongly about. Joy can occur from learning, playing music, and singing. Many times senior citizens feel a sense of joy caring for an animal. Of course, tremendous joy can be experienced from being an involved parent. Many people feel a great sense of joy participating in a sport or activity. Close relationships, family, and the feelings of community can bring joy to people's lives. Begin to write a list of the things that bring joy to your life. Be willing to think about other things that might bring joy to your life. Imagine, as you are participating in your healing and wellness, feeling the joy that manifests from those activities and discovering the positive results in your life. Here are some things on my list.

I feel joy when I am:

1. Serving others
2. Playing guitar and ukulele
3. Writing songs and working on this book
4. Dancing
5. Playing tennis
6. Being outside in the sunlight and nature

7. Gazing at the ocean and sitting on the beach
8. Teaching others about holistic healing and wellness
9. Being with friends and family
10. Being in the wonderful relationship with my sweetheart
11. Spending time with my children
12. Stretching and exercising
13. Hiking in nature and gazing at mountains
14. Having intimate communication and conversations

CHAPTER 11

KINDNESS

REGARDLESS OF SOMEONE'S religion, race, nationality, or philosophy, kindness is a quality that is an essential aspect of healing. Kindness not only helps heal ourselves but also helps bring more healing to the world. As we are exploring all these ingredients of health, one can observe that, like baking a cake, there are many ingredients, yet none are that difficult or impossible to obtain. The acts of kindness in our life ultimately come from a compassionate, healing heart. As we begin each day, regardless of how challenging the day may be, we might consider asking ourselves, "Can I be at least kind today in all my interactions with people and animals?" When people receive an act of kindness, it has the possibility of changing their attitude and even sometimes their life.

When we are angry with someone in the workplace or with a family member, it is important to remember the quality of kindness. There are healthy ways of managing and healing our upsets, which are explored in this book, yet learning to be kind regardless of differences we may have with others is crucial to our own healing. Too often in relationships we either stop communicating or develop an attitude of self-righteousness or judgment when we disagree. Being kind is not pretending to be kind. Being and becoming kind is a muscle that needs development like any other muscle. It is only in changing ourselves rather than trying to change others that we realize the depth of understanding healing and letting go of resignation. Each day can begin with the question, "How and where can I be kind today?"

Healthy Experiment for the Day

How many acts of kindness did I manifest today?

What was the outcome of being more kind throughout the day?

Simple Acts of Kindness

1. Sharing your appreciation with others
2. Saying a simple thank-you
3. Paying attention to others and truly listening when they are speaking
4. Speaking respectfully
5. Respecting other people's time
6. Acknowledging store managers and employees
7. Being considerate and caring
8. Sharing one thing you appreciate about each person you see today.

We all love reading about some act of kindness in the paper or on the Internet. Sometimes I try to understand that person and what inspired him or her to simply help a stranger or an injured animal. Sometimes we see stories of animals helping humans or other animals in a challenging situation. We all feel inspired when we witness these acts of random kindness. When we see an animal acting more humane than humans, that in itself should awaken and inspire us all to be better and healthier as we navigate through our lives.

CHAPTER 12

LOVE

LOVE IS A powerful healer. Many studies have shown that when people experience more love in their life, their capacity for healing and health is greater. Love is a sacred quality in all of us. There is an essential need and desire to give love as well as receive love. The very nature of learning to love ourselves is the most essential quality to our real health insurance. Loving ourselves is not so easy. It is a process of self-development and of self-acceptance. The very relationship we have with ourselves is at the core of our vitality, success, creativity, and continued learning, growing, and healing. The relationship we have with ourselves follows the same guidelines we have with other relationships. Respect, appreciation, gratitude, healthy communication, trust, visions, and goals are all part of the matrix of vibrant health. People feel better about themselves when they keep their promises to themselves. When we deceive ourselves or do not meet the goals we have set forth, we begin to lose faith in ourselves and continue to judge ourselves harshly. Self-judgment, feeling unworthy, feeling unloved, and feeling unlovable become part of a crippling disease affecting us physically and emotionally. Our thoughts about ourselves directly and immediately affect our immune system and nervous system, the two systems of our body that influence everything from the cellular level to the conscious level.

Often people feel their best when they are caring for something else, be it person, pet or plant unconditionally. Just watch people with infants or pets, and you will discover things about those people you never witnessed before. It seems that love flows without hesitation or screening with infants and pets. The quality that is present in both

44

situations is the feeling of full and total acceptance. It is as if people feel that they can be totally free to be themselves without any concern or anxiety of being judged or criticized. When people feel this magic feeling, it almost miraculously opens their heart to give more love. It is as if there is an infinite creative source of love that never tires when this feeling is experienced. The essence of this allows us to discover how important this truly is for our overall well-being and aging with grace. When we feel more accepted in each and every relationship we are in, we automatically open our hearts to give more. The more we give, the better we feel about ourselves. The better we feel about ourselves, the healthier we become. If a heart could talk, it would indeed say, "Yes, I am much happier now feeling loved and giving love, rather than feeling afraid, fearful, and angry." This can be witnessed in every relationship. If one desired a healthy, intimate relationship, the secret would be to first continue to love yourself so that you were able and willing to bring love to someone else in the form of appreciation and acceptance.

Imagine if someone was sharing with you each day things he or she appreciated about you, and you simply felt the person's acceptance and love. My guess is that you would desire to bring even more love through your actions and deeds to that person. Even in the workplace, people perform better and feel healthier at the end of the day when they are working in an atmosphere of love and appreciation. We have all heard the saying "the more you give, the more you receive," but it is the giving without expectations, without strings attached. It is the type of giving in which at the end of the day, we feel better about ourselves. It is in that moment we may hear a voice inside that says, "I am loving myself more and more and appreciating the person I am being and becoming." When we love ourselves, it becomes natural to learn, grow, and change from unhealthy habits to healthy lifestyles. It becomes natural to eat healthier, exercise, learn from emotional wounds, and participate in the process of becoming a healthier person each day. What seemed difficult almost instantly becomes effortless. As we experience our own feelings of love, we become more connected to our true, powerful self. It is as if we have just been reborn and awakened.

LOVING OURSELVES

Loving ourselves does not mean we are perfect. It means we are working on accepting ourselves without self-judgment and, most important, no longer allowing other people's judgment to affect us either.

I had met Glenda at a party where she was teaching belly dancing. Her joy and her love of the art of belly dancing lit up the room. She truly radiated a unique beauty from the inside out. When I spoke with her later in the evening, she shared with me an insightful story that I have never forgotten. She said that she was in a wonderful relationship with someone, but one day the person told her that he truly loved her, but he had a difficult time with her being overweight. Glenda listened compassionately and then very lovingly said, "So what are going to do about your problem?" As Glenda shared this with me, I had an amazing breakthrough regarding myself. Every time I had shared some judgment that I had toward someone else, the problem was truly mine, not theirs. When we love ourselves, we no longer have to feel defensive, protective, or reactive. Since Glenda already loved herself, she no longer had to feel ashamed or defensive about her weight. Though Glenda still could be taking actions to lose weight if she desired, it was not to receive acceptance or love from someone else.

When we love ourselves, we don't make other people's problems ours.

CHAPTER 13

MEDITATION

MEDITATION IS THE art of listening to the voice that speaks through the silence of our prayer or focused centering. Learning to meditate is a tool to assist ourselves to truly relax. When we learn to meditate, the immediate outcome can lower blood pressure, reduce stress, relax muscles, and help us feel more centered, feel guided toward specific actions, and feel reconnected to our spiritual power. In a world that seems to be moving faster and faster, learning to meditate is even more essential for our well-being. Sadly, every day people feel like they just don't have time to take care of their health. We are busy at home, busy at work, challenged by finances, and challenged in relationships, and our health continues to decline when we do not make the time for our health.

Learning to meditate is like setting the internal compass so it aligns with the true purpose and visions of our life. I often share with my patients that meditation and prayer are truly two parts of a whole. While prayer is the speaking part of communication, meditation is the listening part of communication. Too often in relationships, we are better at the talking aspect than the listening. How often have we thought someone is not hearing us, someone is really not listening to what we are saying? Yet when we feel someone really is listening, it almost creates a magical experience. Our relationship with a higher force, a creator, or God follows the same spiritual law of learning to quiet our thoughts so that we can truly hear a divine message if it is being shared with us. Meditation, like prayer, should be a practice that is used each day. Learning to destress is a vital ingredient for our health and continued abundant wellness. There are many ways to learn to meditate, but most important, meditating can be easy as well as fun. There also can be two types of meditating: passive meditation and active meditation.

Three-Minute or Passive Meditation

1. Find a peaceful place either inside or outside where you will not be disturbed.
2. Sit in a relaxed, comfortable position.
3. Close your eyes and tune into a gentle, slow breathing pattern.
4. Focus on a peaceful light, peaceful thoughts, or the grace of divine spirit.
5. Focus on your heart opening to love and guidance.
6. Simply enjoy the quietness and the stillness, letting go of any stressful thoughts with each deep breath.
7. Do this for at least three minutes each day until it becomes easier to quiet the mind and feel the connectedness of your body, mind, and spirit.
8. The more consistent this becomes in your life, the more you will discover allowing yourself to delve deeper and deeper into your own stillness and sacred space.

Active Meditation

This is the art of practicing meditation while participating in an activity. Many times gardeners, hikers, runners, musicians, and healers will share that while they are doing their physical activity, they sometimes feel a shift within themselves appear. The gardener may feel a sacred connection to the earth, the hiker walking through the woods may feel the profound connection to nature, the runner may begin to experience a runner's high as all stress seems to diminish, and the healer may feel the divine experience of oneness working on another person. Each of us as we practice the art of meditation can learn to empower this skill with any activity at any time. In any given moment, something stressful in our lives can shift, becoming the possibility of peace, compassion, love, forgiveness, and hope when we open our hearts.

I am an active tennis player, which I have termed Zen Tennis when I am on the tennis courts. When I am in the zone, my body and mind are working effortlessly and being engaged more effectively in the match. I am more relaxed, yet more energized; I move effortlessly; my instincts are more precise; the ball moves slower as my reactions are quicker and more focused; and most important, I am having more fun and playing at my best.

CHAPTER 14

NUTRITION

THERE ARE HUNDREDS of books about healthy eating and television specials sharing the importance of proper nutrition for preventing disease and creating optimum wellness. Yet approximately 75 percent of the population continues to eat unhealthy, consuming processed fast food and artificial drinks disguised to be healthy. But what is most disturbing is that our leading health profession continues to supply people with more medication without taking the time to explain the essential necessity of eating healthy and proper nutrition to their patients. The very essence of this book is for all of us as a community to understand that the expense of disease will continue to become greater as people are not guided to healthier lifestyles. Of course, we know we cannot make people change, but as doctors, health professionals, and therapists, we have to do our part by being consistent in the message of healing and wellness. Throughout this book I continue to share how often people can be resistant to change, yet when we do change, transformation can occur in our lives. Change is a natural process of learning, growing, and spiritually developing. Learning and beginning to eat better on a daily basis does not have to be difficult. When parents eat healthy, then children are also educated and raised in a healthy environment understanding the importance and the difference between healthy food and the junk food that is advertised to us throughout the day.

SIMPLE, BASIC NUTRITIONAL STRATEGIES

1. Begin eating a healthy breakfast. This can be yogurt, fruit, and nuts; oatmeal with fruit and nuts; a veggie scramble with fruit;

or even a healthy smoothie with almond or coconut milk with banana, berries, apple, or other fruits you desire. You can even make a green drink with veggies. You may add whey or hemp protein powder or veggie protein for additional protein.

2. Have a healthy lunch. This can be tuna salad, chicken salad, or a vegetable salad with avocado. Begin thinking of eating four or five colors of fruit and vegetables each day.

3. Have a healthy dinner. If you eat chicken, fish, turkey, or red meat, be certain to have a larger portion of vegetables with it. It can be steamed broccoli, kale, beans, asparagus, or cabbage. Have assorted vegetables in a fresh salad, leafy green lettuce, spinach, purple cabbage, purple onions, carrots, sprouts, radish, beets, avocadoes, peppers, tomatoes, almonds, or pumpkin seeds. Make your salads colorful and fun.

Begin drinking good water throughout the day and having healthy snacks like cut-up apples, carrots, celery, raisins, almonds, and grapes.

The more you eat healthy, the easier it will become to let go of the unhealthy foods that are loaded with unhealthy sugar, salt, chemicals, and unhealthy fat.

CHAPTER 15

OPPORTUNITY/OPENNESS

OPPORTUNITIES OCCUR IN people's lives more often then we probably realize. An opportunity can create a possibility we didn't even know could exist. There are many types of opportunities, but the opportunities I am sharing about relate to our overall health and positive success in life. Sometimes we have to be willing to receive the grace of an opportunity by simply not pushing it away. Life can have so many missed opportunities simply by not being open to hearing and listening to what someone else may be sharing with us. Every conversation we have with people can lead to opportunities when we are truly engaged. You never know who you may be talking to who might need your services or whose services you may desire. In essence every success in someone's life began by someone being open and listening sincerely to the opportunity before him or her.

I remember when I was attending a seminar in radiology as a chiropractic student. I was in my last semester and determining what direction I was going to head in when graduating. During that seminar I met another chiropractor who was leading a seminar in another room in the hotel. He was teaching chiropractors the importance of educating their patients once they became doctors. This doctor, a leader in the chiropractic profession, began sharing with me the importance of working for another successful chiropractor before starting my own office. Thankfully, I was open to his wisdom and greeted this opportunity of our meeting as a blessing. I followed his recommendations and was thankful each day I did. When we are open, opportunities change our lives forever in a powerful way.

Questions

1. Can you think of opportunities that occurred in your life?
2. Can you remember the people who changed your life when you were open to what they shared with you?
3. Imagine someone telling you to see a holistic chiropractor for a health condition you were having. Would you be open and follow their recommendation?

CHAPTER 16

PEACE

How do we find peace within ourselves in a world that is not always at peace? Becoming more peaceful is a skill we have to learn. As we learn to become more at peace, we bring peacefulness wherever we go. So many people are on medication for anxiety and depression. Patients will share with me that often their medical doctor will not even ask what challenges or stresses they are facing in life. Instead, the doctor begins writing prescriptions for them to feel better without addressing what is causing the disharmony in someone's life. For each of us, life can be challenging. We all have to discover ways to bring more peace into our lives and activities that reconnect us to our higher consciousness. For some it can be prayer and meditation. For others it is walking through the woods or hiking. It can come in the form of playing music, singing, or dancing. As we are expressing our creative spirit, we feel a deeper sense of peace inside. In truth we feel better about ourselves when we feel more accepting of ourselves, more self-loving, and are pursuing goals in healthy ways. Peace is a feeling, but it resides in the actions we take. Reminding ourselves to breathe deeply and feel the breath of life instantly creates physiological ease throughout our body.

I was recently at my sweetheart's mother's home. Carolyn is a master weaver on a loom. She has been weaving since early childhood. When she weaves I can see the peaceful healing energy coming through her. She weaves these beautiful chenille scarves, which I have termed "Soul Scarfs," since each beautiful scarf resonates with each person's spirit. She has taught me how to weave on the loom as well. It is amazing how

I can sit there for several hours watching a "Soul Scarf" come to life in this sacred, peaceful, creative space.

In a world that struggles to find peace, we have to discover how to bring peace to our own immediate family. So often families are in their own turmoil facing so many challenges. Creating peace begins with healthy communication. Each person has their own position that they feel right and righteous about. The bridge to peaceful communication is developing the art of compassionate listening. Through learning the process of everyday healing, we discover that peace is obtainable when we change ourselves for the better first. In relationships we do not always have to agree, but we can discover healthy communication to allow each person's view to be expressed. When we begin to discover the art of healthy, peaceful communication in our families, we can build a bridge to a healthier world.

GIVE PEACE A CHANCE

1. How can you bring more peace to your own family?
2. How can you feel more peaceful at work?
3. Do you feel at peace in your intimate relationship?
4. How can you see yourself feeling more at peace with yourself?
5. For one day imagine not trying to prove something to someone else, not defending something about yourself, and not wishing people were different from the way they were. Imagine how that might feel to you.

CHAPTER 17

QUESTIONS

CHILDREN INTUITIVELY ALWAYS ask questions. As adults, too often we have forgotten to ask questions, especially when it comes to our overall health. Here are essential questions we should all be asking when seeing doctors for ourselves or others.

1. What is causing this pain or condition?
2. What can be done to correct or prevent this problem?
3. What are the side effects of this medication? How long will I need to be taking it? Will the problem improve with the medication?
4. How will these treatments help this condition?
5. Are there any complications that can occur from this surgery?
6. What is necessary to prevent the problems that members in my family have?
7. What can I do to become healthier physically, emotionally, and nutritionally?
8. What is causing these symptoms? (Headaches, allergies, indigestion, asthma, colic, pain, difficulty sleeping, anxiety, feeling depressed, fatigue, dizziness.)
9. When undergoing any surgery or therapy for a condition, always ask when you will be able to work or play again in optimum capacity.
10. What can I do to prevent and reverse arthritis, diabetes, high blood pressure, or colitis?

OUR REAL HEALTH INSURANCE A-Z AND MORE

Never accept answers to questions that sound like clichés.

1. It is just a normal childhood condition.
2. It is just a hereditary condition.
3. It is just stress.
4. It is just part of aging.

One day when Derek was receiving his adjustment for his low back he said that he noticed children in the office. He mentioned that his daughter suffered with asthma since she was a few months old. He said over the last five years he had to bring her to the hospital a few times when she was having an asthma attack. He asked me if I treated children with health problems. The answer was yes. On the next visit Derek brought his beautiful daughter to the office. I explained to her how we were going to try to help her, and if she would be willing to make some changes in her eating patterns. She agreed she would. After receiving four to six adjustments to help balance the nervous system, eating healthier and avoiding toxic food, and practicing appropriate breathing exercises, she was feeling better, having more energy, and breathing effortlessly. She continued to improve, and her medical doctors were able to reduce all the medication she was taking.

One question from her dad led to changing that little girl's life forever.

CHAPTER 18

REST/RELATIONSHIPS

REST

TAKING THE TIME to rest is essential for our overall well-being. Resting is taking a break from the normal activities and giving the body and the mind a chance to disengage from the daily stress. Resting can be curling up with a good book on a hammock on a sunny day. It can be going for a nice walk in the park and sitting by a river or lake. It could be taking a drive and going away for the day and visiting a waterfall. Resting can be even taking a nap if you have not been getting enough sleep. Rest can be different for different people, but the purpose is to turn the busy mind off and be okay with doing nothing in particular other than enjoying the moment.

REST TO DESTRESS

1. What do you do to rest in your life?
2. How do you feel when you do nothing and simply rest?
3. Do you allow yourself to take a nap if you are tired?
4. Do you have a strategy in your life to rest?

Relationships

The relationships in our lives are the mirror for us to truly see ourselves. Each relationship can serve as a measure of how we are learning and evolving as a healthy person. So often in our lives we are either judging others or feeling judged. As we truly follow the everyday healing guidance throughout this book, we discover our own relationship with ourselves improving. Almost like magic, as we improve ourselves, we feel more compassionate, more understanding, more loving, and less defensive and guarded. Over the years I have witnessed so many of my patients discover new, healthy relationships with the most important people in their lives when they focused on changing themselves rather than trying to change others. My own life has been a testimony of this as well as I navigated through the battleground of divorce, where at times it felt impossible to see the light at the end of the tunnel. Healing takes us on a journey, and when we are willing, transformation can occur in our lives. My own story about my divorce is shared in my memoir, *Divorce: An Uncommon Love Story*. So often in the most precious relationships in our lives, we are feeling guarded, overreacting, being defensive, trying to prove something, or being resigned or controlling. When we heal ourselves and surrender these old dysfunctional mechanisms, a new world opens up to us with magical opportunities for unconditional love.

Relationship Exercise

1. Think of one significant person in your life where you feel stressed.
2. What is the emotion or feeling that you have regarding the circumstance with this person? Do you feel upset, frustrated, sad, or angry?
3. When you tend to feel these emotions or thoughts, what do you tend to do? What is your typical behavior? Do you verbalize it, do you share what you feel in a healthy way, do you stop speaking to

the person, do you pretend that nothing is wrong, or do you wait for the other person to say something?

4. If it was an intimate partner, son, daughter, brother, or sister, how long would you go without addressing this circumstance?
5. How does this behavior make you feel?
6. How do you think it affects your health?

Often we get stuck in old-brain thinking and patterns, waiting on other people to change so that our life can improve. Most of us might spend our entire life trying to change the people we care about, causing more and more frustration in the relationship. The only person we can change is ourselves!

1. What do I want to create regarding my relationship with this person?
2. I am willing to see how I have been either reacting, defending, being resigned, or pretending in this relationship.
3. I am now ready to accept my own responsibility for keeping myself stuck and blaming the other person.
4. I am ready to apologize where appropriate for any of my own behaviors and share what I truly desire in the relationship.
5. As I am healing myself, I can see and understand that if I want healthier communication, to feel more honored and respected, and to feel more appreciated, I first have to become the deliverer of what I desire and become more respectful and more loving.

CHAPTER 19

SLEEP/STRESS

SLEEP

SADLY, SO MANY people take medication to help them sleep. Having a restful sleep is essential for the body to recuperate from our busy, active day. One of the first symptoms I want to see improve when I am working on patients is them sleeping better. If we sleep better, all other ailments will improve quicker. When we do not sleep well, it is almost guaranteed that the day will be more stressful. So how do you begin to sleep better if you are having difficulty? We have to learn how to relax and turn down the volume of business and noise going on in our brain. The world we live in can be very stressful. Most people watch stimulating television shows before they go to sleep, which further activates the busy brain. One of my patients had difficulty sleeping for years. If she was lucky, she would get two hours a night sleeping. Her life has been very challenging, and over the years she had developed unhealthy habits prior to going to sleep. When she began doing some of the exercises below, her sleeping patterns immediately changed for the better.

HEALTHY HABITS BEFORE GOING TO SLEEP

1. Take five minutes to stretch and undo the stresses of the day.
2. Take at least three minutes for prayer or meditation time to empty the mind of stressful thoughts.

3. Read inspirational material before bedtime until you become sleepy.

4. Listen to meditative music or a guided meditative relaxing program to assist in learning how to disengage from the day.

Stress

Another word for stress can be life. There will always be stress, and there has always been stress. Often people become stressed when unexpected bad things occur, but also when good things are occurring like building a new home, starting a new job, planning a wedding, going on a date, or meeting new people. In essence we bring our own stress wherever we go. Life will never stop being stressful, but as we change ourselves, how we respond to the stress of life will change significantly. Instead of making ourselves sick, we will discover our own mind and body becoming healthier.

Strategies for Reducing Unhealthy Stress

1. Identify what you are feeling stressed about.
2. Become clear of the emotions you are feeling and be okay with what you are feeling at the moment.
3. Ask yourself if these emotions and responses to the stress are healthy and helpful regarding the situation.
4. Take the time to meditate about the circumstance and ask for inner guidance.
5. Write down some specific actions you can take to create a healthier outcome with this challenging time.
6. Take the time to do something playful or fun.
7. Seek out assistance from wellness coaches if you feel hopeless and stuck.
8. Regardless of what you may feel stressed about, pause and observe what you are grateful for in your life. Take the time to acknowledge yourself for accomplishments you have obtained during stressful times.

CHAPTER 20

THOUGHT/THINKING

OUR REAL HEALTH insurance is how we think about our health. If we think that our health is truly one of the most important aspects of our life, then there will be specific actions that align with those thoughts. Everyone says they want to be healthy, yet in the world we live in, most of us have been taught how to be sick. After a while we begin believing that we don't have the time to take care of our health or cannot afford to take care of our health. The first thing that changes when we begin to become healthier is the process of reconnecting to loving ourselves enough to make changes in our life that empower what we truly desire.

I have so many patients who are already on medication for high blood pressure and diabetes, yet they are still not changing any of the unhealthy habits in their life. They have been seeing medical doctors who continue to prescribe more and more medication without taking the time to explain the necessity of eating healthier and exercising every day. All these patients tell me that they desire to become healthier. They say they are trying to change, they say that they know they need to change, but something has not clicked into their brain yet. Sadly, when the very doctors they see do not explain the consequences of taking more and more medication without changing their lifestyle, these patterns continue and are passed on to their children and grandchildren. Most patients simply begin to believe if they don't feel any significant amount of pain, the medication is helping these diseases from degenerating further. When I begin to explain these conditions to my patients, and the serious side effects of the medication they have been taking for years, and how their own body has been measurably losing function, they begin to understand for the first time that their health can improve. If I can help people think differently about their own vitality and possible vibrant health, the path of assisting those people to greater health and well-being is 95 percent easier. Often when I explain how our body works and the difference between masking a symptom with medication and discovering what is causing a problem and correcting the problem, a patient will say, "That makes perfect sense."

Imagine if we had a leak dripping water into the kitchen. The first thing we would do is get a bucket to catch the water to protect the floor. We would be correctly reacting to the crisis. But if we never addressed what was causing the leak and continued to get more buckets as the problem continued, eventually we would be facing a major, very expensive problem. In this analogy the buckets are the drugs we take for the symptoms, which have a purpose, but the purpose was never to correct the problem or become a lifestyle while we ignored what was truly causing the condition.

Every thought we have has a physiological reaction in our body. If you think of a juicy bright lemon right now and begin to see yourself bite into the lemon, you might already sense the saliva in your mouth changing. There is no real lemon present, but the real thought of a lemon immediately causes a physiological response. Now imagine if you are happy about something, or you are holding on to anger or frustration. Each thought will affect our health in various ways. Many times frustrated thoughts are subconscious below our conscious awareness and continue to rob our body of energy and vitality all day long.

Questions

1. How do you think about your own health, and what strategies do you have that align with those thoughts?
2. Do you think you could become healthier if you changed certain habits and improved on what you were already doing?

3. If you take medication, how long have you been taking it, and do you know the side effects it can cause?
4. Do you think you understand what arthritis is, or diabetes, or high blood pressure, if you have any of these diseases?
5. What do you tell yourself when you know you should change certain unhealthy habits yet continue to do them?
6. If you really felt excited about your life and good about yourself, what, if anything, do you think you would change?
7. If you were facing a serious health crisis, what, if anything, do you think you would change?
8. How do you feel about yourself when you know you are making changes to become healthier and more fulfilled in your life?

I have known so many patients through the years who either thought that they were addicted to certain behaviors or felt it was just too difficult to change habits they have had for so many years. Yet most of us when faced with a crisis will immediately change. Maybe you have known friends or family members who smoked every day, then were diagnosed with lung cancer, and then stopped smoking. Many people when faced with dialysis will have no other alternative than changing their eating behavior if they want to continue living. Let's not wait for a crisis to change how we think and the actions we take regarding our health and our life.

CHAPTER 21

UNDERSTANDING

Throughout this book there are the qualities that are necessary to become healthier in our lives. Yet without true understanding it becomes difficult to achieve the goals we desire. Everyone wants to be healthy and prevent disease, yet continue to do the very things that can lead to disease and not do many of the things consistently to discover more vitality and wellness in our lives. We know we should eat healthier, yet struggle with making those required changes. We know we should exercise yet to often find reasons to not find or make the time to integrate healthy routines in our life.

In my initial consultation with a patient I take the time to explain what may be causing the problem that the patient is having. So many of the patients share with me about the doctors they have seen, and the medications they are taking. Many patients have already been diagnosed with high blood pressure, diabetes, or arthritis, yet do not have a significant understanding about the disease. Too often people have recurrent back problems and can easily assume it is because of their jobs, or the process of aging. As I begin to explain to them about their problem I often hear someone say, "I never thought about it like that before." "That makes perfect sense."

I believe if all doctors took the time to explain to patients starting with parents in regards to their children we would begin to see disease reduced, and wellness increased in people's lives. The necessity of medication would decrease, as people understood the importance of making changes in their lives to correct and prevent conditions from becoming worse.

Throughout the years I have referred patients to other specialists to rule out certain problems, as well as hear what their recommendations were. I have had the benefit of knowing excellent neurosurgeons, and orthopedic doctors when I thought back surgery might be necessary for my patients. These doctors also sat in the same room as me as many experts in the field spoke about the value of conservative chiropractic treatment and other therapies before a patient was recommended for back surgery. When I am referred a patient by medical doctors I am hopeful that our health care system is understanding the importance of all doctors and therapists working together to assist people to greater health.

As doctors take the time to understand about each other, as insurance companies take the time to understand holistic approaches to health problems, I am certain the cost of health care for all of us can come down measurably. "Our real health insurance" is available to everyone regardless of age, income, location, or education.

ASK THE QUESTIONS TO UNDERSTAND

1. What is causing my child's asthma, or allergies?
2. What is causing my child's learning disabilities?
3. What is causing my headaches?
4. What is causing my back pain?
5. What is causing my tooth to hurt?
6. What is causing my stomach pain and infrequent bowel movements?
7. What is causing my high blood pressure, arthritis, or diabetes?
8. What is causing my anxiety or depression?
9. What can be done medically and naturally to prevent or reverse these health conditions?

CHAPTER 22

VISION

VISION IS ESSENTIAL for ongoing healing and wellness in our lives. Often I ask my patients what they desire regarding their health when I first consult with them. Most will say they want to feel better, and they will do anything to get out of the pain they are feeling. When I ask them what they desire after that, most people look confused. In essence most people when it comes to health do not have a vision beyond just, "Please get me feeling better." Let's face it; that is how the medical and drug community has trained us our whole life. Haven't we all heard, "Pop, pop, fizz, fizz, oh, what a relief it is"? But real health is what we do after we feel better. What would you be doing that you have not done, if you felt better? Everything each of us has achieved in life has been initiated by a vision. Whether it was learning to ride a bike or a desire to finish school, make the baseball team, or be a talented artist or successful businessperson, all required a vision that moved us through each challenge we faced. Without a clear, powerful vision, we give up before we even give ourselves a true opportunity to discover what is possible. Sometimes we can learn a great deal from children or remembering when we were a child.

Think back when you were learning to ride a bike and how often you fell. Maybe dozens of times you even scraped your knees and felt the pain from the bike landing on top of you, yet you never gave up. You may have wanted to at the moment when you saw your knee bleeding, and you began yelling and crying, but you didn't. You may have never thought about it, but the reason was that you had a clear vision of what riding that bike meant to you. Perhaps it meant feeling older, freedom, getting places faster, speed, and having fun. Well, your body is your new bike. Unless you have a vision of what it means to become healthier, to have more energy, to feel emotionally healthier, to lose those extra pounds, to prevent illness, and to prevent health conditions from getting worse, your health will just continue to decline.

CREATING A VISION

1. What is the vision you desire for your physical health?
2. If you were physically healthier, what would you like to do better, or do again? Maybe walking, playing tennis or golf, riding a bike, working in the garden, going back to work, or working without limitations.
3. What is your vision for your nutritional well-being? If you were eating healthier every day, how would that make you feel? If you had more energy, lost weight, and discovered your high blood pressure and diabetes improving, how would that begin to change your life?
4. What is your vision for the relationships in your life—your significant other, the relationships with your children, your family, and your friends? Imagine a vision where all these relationships improved and you discovered healthier communication, more understanding, more compassion, and the experience of true love. How would you feel about yourself if you were becoming healthier emotionally and understood there was only one person we could change in our lives, and that was ourselves? Yet when we did, all relationships improved, and most important our life improved.
5. Imagine if you had a vision to make a powerful contribution to the world.
6. Begin to write down your visions in all these areas of your life. Be clear, be specific, and then write down what actions you are ready to take to achieve these goals.

———— ⌒ ————

CHAPTER 23

Wow Walking

Wow walking is something most of us can begin doing today. We all know that walking is very healthy for our body. Different from running, it is easy on the joints, so it is available for anyone. But wow walking is different from just walking, or walking to increase your heart rate. Wow walking is taking the time to reconnect with nature and the miraculous world we live in. We are all so busy in our lives, thinking of all the things we need to do, which continuously activates stress to our body and mind. Wow walking is ideal on a nature trail or in a park, but it can be anywhere. Slow, relaxed breathing is essential during a wow walk. Breathe in oxygen, feeling life filter into your body, and breathe out carbon dioxide, which is letting go of all the stress we are carrying around. Wow walking is like a vacation for our body and mind. As you are walking with this peaceful pattern of breathing, begin to notice and observe the beauty of nature around you. Listen to the musical song of the birds, and pretend you are able to understand their enchanting language. Observe the trees and flowers, the various shapes and colors, and behold the miracle of this creative force of life. Pause to consider the miracle of life that exists through the changing seasons as you breathe. At some moment you will hear a voice inside yourself that says, "Wow." Now you are wow walking.

As you continue to walk, look up to the clouds and sky, allowing your own mind and heart to imagine all the blessings in your own life and the excitement in your life as you are pursuing your new visions to become healthier in mind, body, and spirit. Every day make wow walking part of your healing strategies connecting to the magnificence of your life and life itself. Wow walking reminds us who we really are and what is possible if we reconnect to our own spiritual power. The simple act of wow walking can reduce high blood pressure; diminish physical and emotional stress from our body; increase blood flow to our muscles and joints to reduce and prevent arthritis; enhance neurological activity and blood flow to our brain to improve creativity, vitality, and memory; and most important, have us feel better about ourselves physically and emotionally.

REMINDERS WHEN WOW WALKING

1. Breathe slowly.
2. Surrender to the beauty and magic of nature.
3. If the flowers and trees had a voice, what do you think they might share with you?
4. Feel the wind on your skin. What is the wind sharing with you?
5. As you are wow walking, begin to see what you are ready to change in your life to improve.
6. Take the time thinking about all the important relationships in your life, and see those people surrounded by light and love.
7. As you look up to the sky, what message might the sky that holds the infinite galaxies share with you?

CHAPTER 24

X Factor

THE X FACTOR is that which is hard to understand with our logical mind. The X factor is that which we cannot know when we begin or engage in participating with our healing and ongoing wellness. We do not know how much better we can become until we commit to the process, have a vision of an outcome, and take the actions that are necessary. We all want the quick fix, and we want results quickly without investing much time or money in the pursuit of what we say we desire. The X factor is an experience that occurs after we have been applying all the guidelines as a lifestyle and then discover that aspects of our life improve beyond which we could have dreamed or contemplated. It is when a patient says to me, "I could not have imagined I would be feeling this good again and doing the things I love again."

In the area of relationships, so often people will share how the relationship with their son or daughter or their intimate partner has transformed since they have been healing themselves. The X factor is a miraculous place, though seldom visited by most people, because we have been trained to accept illness and broken relationships as the norm. We have been taught to treat problems from the outside, rather than looking inward to observe the things about ourselves to change. The X factor is the space from which we experience healing, love, and healthy changes. If we were taught to be healthy and how to take care of our health as a lifestyle starting when we were a child, then the X factor would be an ongoing experience, discovering healing and trans-forming as a way of life. Who knows what would be possible for us as spiritual human beings? Who knows what we would be capable of? As amazed as we are of what computers can do and how they are advancing each moment, we would become amazed at what our body and mind was capable of and be excited and in awe of the X factor.

One afternoon I entered the room to adjust one of my patients who was seventy-five years old at the time. Her name is Ms. Harris. She said that she had to share something with me, as well as ask me something before the treatment today. I had no idea what she was going to ask. She had been feeling better since receiving adjustments and had discovered that her arthritic knees and lower back were functioning and moving better than they had in years. That in itself was an x factor for her. But today she looked at me differently, as she asked whether these adjustments could be affecting her womanhood. I laughed and said, "What do you mean?" She said she was feeling like a young girl again and could not understand what was going on in her body. Well, I smiled again and said, "Adjustments and healing don't just work on the parts; it is neurologically affecting your whole body, the whole house. It sounds like your furnace is heating up again." Then we both laughed. But she could never have dreamed that by receiving adjustments, her female aliveness would be coming back. She felt like a schoolgirl again and was ready to find herself a young man. We both couldn't stop laughing that day. We have no idea what is possible when it comes to healing until we are open to receive and take the actions necessary to improve our health.

THE X FACTOR IN YOUR LIFE

Can you think of a time in your life when something wonderful happened that you could not have imagined?

As example in my own life, when I was diagnosed with ulcerative colitis in my early twenties, I was told nothing could be done other than steroids for the rest of my life and that this condition could easily lead to colon cancer. That path would have certainly led to a life of disease and a very different life from the one I have lived. But thankfully, my openness to see a friend's holistic chiropractor and then the willingness to follow his guidelines achieved outcomes I could not have imagined.

1. I never did take any steroids.
2. Within two to three months, I began to feel better than I had felt in the last six months.
3. In about seven to nine months, all the symptoms, including blood in my stool and everyday pain, were gone. My bowel movements became normal again without pain or discomfort.
4. I began to feel physically and emotionally healthier in all aspects of my life.
5. And out of this experience, I decided to become a holistic chiropractor, serving others to greater healing and wellness, rather than pursuing medical school. And from that experience, I continued to make my own physical and emotional health a lifetime journey.

Prior to becoming sick with ulcerative colitis, I had never been to a chiropractor and knew absolutely nothing about the profession. But because of this scenario, an X factor occurred that changed my life forever. I always share with my patients that out of the worst situation in my life, the most amazing miracle manifested. My willingness to be coached and my willingness to change created a shift in my life that altered it forever.

CHAPTER 25

YES

WHEN WE GREET life with a yes, we enter into new possibilities that lead us to deeper abundance and well-being. A simple yes when someone shares something that might assist us with whatever challenge we are facing can change our life. As simple as a yes might seem, we often respond to life with excuses, reasonable explanations to support sabotaging what we truly desire.

Often I meet people who tell me about health problems they have, yet who are resistant to hear about alternatives that can assist them to improve. Instead of greeting the opportunity with a yes, we respond with rational reasons to not even discover what may change our life. For thirty-five years, I have educated my patients on the importance of everyday healing strategies. Like everyone else I can be lazy and resistant to change. I am always looking at and discovering how to make things easier, to attain the goals I want to achieve. So I developed simple exercises that just take a few minutes a day to do yet when done every day have tremendous beneficial results. Becoming healthier is not difficult, but it does require greeting opportunities with a yes.

I met Bob and his wife while staying at an inn in the mountains of North Carolina. The last morning before going home, we shared breakfast together and had an opportunity to talk with each other. I found out that Bob had been a professor at Georgia Tech but sadly had been diagnosed with terminal cancer and had just a few months to live. The coughing I had heard throughout the weekend when we were at the inn now made sense. In the conversation he asked what I did, and I shared that I was a holistic chiropractor. He seemed interested, so I continued explaining about the healing capabilities of the body. Unexpectedly, he said he would like to come to my office and was open to what I might be able to do, even if it was just feeling less pain. He shared he had been through all the radiation therapy and chemotherapy, so medically there was nothing else medical doctors could do.

Bob came into the office that week. I truly was surprised. We both understood that his body had become very weak and very toxic from the cancer as well as all the medications he had been on. But we both knew that there was nothing to lose in this process of healing. As I began to work on Bob, I could tell he was not used to receiving this type of treatment where specific touch and specific breathing patterns were initiated. But after a while, Bob began to relax, and he spontaneously began to shake. When I asked him what he was feeling, he began to open up and share about his life. With tears in his eyes, he shared that when he was four years old, his father died unexpectedly. He was the youngest child with three older sisters. He began to realize as he lay on the chiropractic table that he had to become the man in the house at an early age. In essence he did not feel like he had a childhood, and as he continued to share this story, he continued to cry, sharing with me that he had never remembered crying in his whole life. I saw Bob for another visit in the office the following week, and again his tears began to release emotions that had been stored up in his body his entire life. He had become an intellectual, a professor, successful in his life by most standards, yet he had become disconnected from the little boy who had lost his father at an early age. As he lay on the table, this sixty-three-year-old man appeared like a four-year-old boy, sobbing yet for the first time, healing and releasing the pain that had been held inside his whole life.

Three months later I received a phone call from a young man, who shared that he was one of Bob's sons. He wanted to let me know that Bob had passed on, yet the true reason for his call was to tell me that after his father saw me for those two visits, he was a changed man. He told me that his father shared things with him and his two siblings that he had never shared before. He went on to say that they never truly had a close relationship with their dad until these last few months. For the first time, their dad opened up to all of them, sharing about his own difficulties in life and how much he loved them all. His son went on to say that he just wanted to call me and say thank you. "We don't know what happened in those visits with our dad," he said, "but it made all the difference in the world to all of us."

Being Able to Say Yes without Excuses

1. Are you eating healthier?
2. Are you learning more about your own health?
3. Are you becoming more responsible in your own life?
4. Are you working on the relationships in your life?
5. Are you discovering more ways to have fun in your life?
6. As you are improving your health, are you feeling better about yourself?
7. Are you creating visions in your life to get excited about?
8. Are you seeking out health coaches, therapists, and doctors to assist you on your path of healing and wellness?

CHAPTER 26

ZEN ZONE

REGARDLESS OF RELIGION or belief, experiencing the Zen Zone is being in an enlightened mind. When we are in a Zen state of mind, the choices in our life are more clear and profound. We deeply understand that external pleasures, such as a bigger home, more money, or success, may feel good, but they can never heal our inner self. When we experience Zen, we feel at peace with ourselves, we have self-acceptance, and we feel more loving and accepting of others. Ultimately, healing physically and emotionally is a process of developing a life that feels more meaningful and being fulfilled in every area of your life. You feel you are living in the moment, yet clear on the visions you are evolving toward.

I remember years ago reading about two monks who were traveling on a road when they both saw a mother holding a baby and trying to cross a rushing stream. Without any hesitation one of the monks asked the woman if she needed assistance and carried her across the stream. About a mile down the road, the other monk with a puzzled face asked why he had helped the woman, since in this particular monastery it was improper to touch a woman. The monk replied, "My brother, I put the young woman and her baby down about a mile ago. Why are you still carrying her?"

This is living in the Zen. You respond to life with a clear yes without complicating the simplicity of life. An enlightened being has learned the rules and then lives beyond the rules. Often people find this difficult to understand.

I am reminded of the story of Jesus, when he comes to the aid of Mary Magdalene. Everyone feels righteous, throwing the stones at Mary for being sinful, yet only when Jesus asks them to look inward at their own sins do they pause to reconsider their actions. When we live in the Zen, everything in our life is more at ease. We are balanced, we feel clear, and we feel we are in the spiritual zone.

Part 2
The Emotional Connection to the Most Common Health Conditions

Dr. Marty Finkelstein

Learning Healing Energetic Exercises
Shifting from Old Brain to New Brain

"Everything you have ever seen or learned has cellular imprint. Old hurts, both physical and emotional are stored in your cells."

—Kondis Blakely, MFCC, author of *Your Body Remembers*

When we truly learn to listen to our body, we become more conscious and connected to our life and the lives of others. Learning to listen to the language of the body is like a musician listening to the sounds of his or her instrument. When we appreciate how the wisdom of our body speaks to us, we can begin to discover a deeper level of wellness within ourselves. When our body feels out of balance or stressed, we can begin to hear our innate consciousness attempting to get our attention. When we recognize the most subtle interferences with our energy level and vitality, we can learn to ask ourselves questions that help us discover what emotional core issues can be affecting our health, as well as explore a pathway of generating conscious healthy changes in our lives.

The following are the most common symptoms that affect people each day. Most of these conditions are never addressed from the root cause, and sadly, these problems lead to further illness and disease. Millions of people each day take medication for these symptoms, yet the symptoms are only temporarily masked, requiring people to take then stronger medication as a way of life. After years of continuous medication, people are finally diagnosed with an illness where eventually surgery is recommended. Sometimes after the surgery, even more medication is then required. This is a vicious disease cycle that so many people feel trapped in, and they never realize and understand the concepts of everyday healing.

CHAPTER 27

HEADACHES
(LIGHTHEADEDNESS, DIZZINESS, DISORIENTATION, CONFUSION, HEAD PRESSURE, SPACINESS)

I HAVE PATIENTS who will tell me that they have suffered from headaches their entire life. Headaches have various patterns. Some headaches can be felt along the sides of the head in the temporal region. Another headache may appear toward the top of the head and the parietal region. Some headaches may be felt behind the eyes and toward the back of the head in the occipital region. Many people have been diagnosed with migraine-type headaches, which can be associated with dizziness and nausea. Headaches that are associated with our mucous membranes are referred to as sinus headaches. Headaches may have a diagnostic orientation associated with toxicity, spinal misalignments causing nerve interference, chemical imbalances, and thought and emotional integrity. Some patients have described their head pain as a dull, aching pain, while others have described their headaches as sharp and pounding. When people have headaches for years, they will tend to categorize their headaches, from their normal "I can live with it" headache to "I can't function when my headache is this bad." Regardless of the type of headache and regardless of how often it occurs, it is important to understand that our body is speaking to us in the language of symptoms to bring our attention to our present consciousness. Masking the pain or ignoring the problem would be no different from having a leak dripping from your ceiling and simply getting a bucket to catch the water yet not addressing the cause of the problem. It then can become easy to rationalize that when the ceiling is no longer leaking, the problem has also disappeared.

The purpose of these thought- and emotion-based exercises is to uncover the essence behind the stress we are feeling. We have all been trained to minimize our feelings and suppress what is truly happening in our body. It has become easy to say, "I am stressed because of work, or finances, or my relationship, or my lack of relationship." It is only when we learn to distinguish what we are feeling and how we are truly reacting to the circumstances in our lives that we discover an opportunity to become healthier. Like a person stuck in quicksand, the more you struggle to get out, the deeper you become stuck.

The more we feel stuck in our lives, the more we continue to react the same way, and the more hopeless we feel. Only when we change our paradigm and shift our consciousness can change and transformation occur.

Strategies to Do the Emotional Exercises

1. Make time to have no distractions.
2. Create a comfortable space to be in.
3. Allow yourself to be present and focus sincerely on the questions that are asked.
4. Be willing to be honest and uncensored, allowing for the authentic benefits of the exercise.
5. Take your time, giving yourself permission to feel your body and mind as you are addressing these issues in your life.
6. Feel good about yourself for taking the time to work on becoming healthier in your life.
7. In each exercise you are asked to feel the emotion that has been present in your life. Emotions and feelings are specific. Here are examples of emotions to choose from:

Anger, sadness, fear, frustration, loneliness, confusion, hopelessness, joy, peace, compassion, happiness, excitement, hope, and love.

Headache Energetic Paradigm

1. Ask yourself, why is my head hurting? Where in my life am I feeling pressure, dizzy, confused, or spacey? What is my body attempting to tell me?
2. Have I done anything physically different? Perhaps a new exercise regimen?
3. Have I been eating healthy food or junk food?
4. What have I been thinking or feeling?

My head has been hurting because I have been feeling pressure or confused about _____ (specific stress).

When I feel this pressure related to this stress, I begin to feel _____ (specific emotion).

When I feel _____ I tend to _____ (specific action).

After I do that, I then feel _____.

Typically, before I get a headache, I feel tension around my _____ (part of body).

When my head hurts, I can feel other parts of my body become _____.

What I usually do when my head hurts is _____.

What I usually do when I feel these thoughts and emotions is _____.

When my head hurts, my energy level tends to _____.

When my head is hurting, I am more _____ in personal relationships.

As we allow ourselves to explore these thoughts and feelings, we begin to discover the underlying core issues that are affecting our health and our life. These answers usually will be present very quickly, because they are already in our subconscious just like information stored in the memory of a computer. It is particularly important to observe how our typical headache, which so often we rationalize, can and does affect every relationship we are in. As we avoid observing the probable causes of our symptoms, we diminish the vibrant energy in our body as well as the passion, love, and compassion in our partnerships.

The next part of the exercise is creating healing and new possibilities for our wellness. The answers to these questions are not stored in our subconscious. Instead it is like having a fresh canvas in front of you, where you can explore and playfully discover what you want to create.

When I am feeling pressure or confusion in my life related to _____, I would like to create _____ (be specific with a feeling) instead of my usual patterns of reacting to these stresses.

If I was creating that, in my life I would begin to feel _____ (be specific).

How that would affect my energy and relationships is _____ (be specific).

I can imagine that if I became more conscious of my body, thoughts, and feelings that my health and my life would _____.

When I begin to feel stress and pressure in my life, I am now going to _____.

When we first begin to do these wellness emotional exercises, it can be more difficult than we realize. Like any exercise we have to learn to be consistent and apply the exercise the correct way. The more we begin working these new muscles, the stronger we become, and more important, we begin to feel better about ourselves.

This is an example of how this exercise can be completed with the willingness to explore our thoughts and feelings.

My head has been hurting because I have been thinking of all the things I need to do at work. When I think about all these things, particularly the things I do not like to do, I begin to feel overwhelmed, depressed, and confused. When I feel overwhelmed, depressed, and confused, I begin to think that I am not capable, and I begin to think it is hopeless. When my head hurts, I feel even more frustrated. Typically, before my head hurts, I feel tension around my neck and shoulders becoming tighter and stiff. When my head hurts, I can feel other parts of my body become restricted, tight, and painful. What I usually do when my head hurts is retreat in a cave and want to be left alone and numb the pain. What I usually do when I feel these thoughts and emotions is suppress them and not want to think about them. When my head hurts, my energy level becomes diminished. When my head is hurting, I become more irritable, unavailable, upset, critical, and impatient in intimate relationships.

What I truly want to create instead of having headaches and feeling bad is to become healthier, have more energy, feel excited about my life, and not feel like my head is "constipated." If I was creating that in my life, I would begin to feel more alive and better about myself and everyone I was participating with in my life. I want to create a more joyful atmosphere with my work and become more organized so that I do not feel so overwhelmed. I believe if I did this, I would begin to feel hopeful and inspired again. If I was creating this in my life, I could see how my intimate relationships would only improve and how my energy level would become greater. I can see that if I became more conscious of my health and my life, everything would have the possibility of improving.

CHAPTER 28

DIGESTIVE DISORDERS
(GUT FEELING, HOLDING IN, EATING ME UP, HOLDING ON TO, PRESSURE, UPSET, IRRITABILITY)

PEOPLE TAKE ALL types of medication to ease the discomforts from abdominal stress. There are a host of symptoms, such as bloating, gas, pressure, belching, constipation, diarrhea, and pain, that can lead to a number of disorders like irritable bowel syndrome, acid reflux, colitis, diverticulitis, ulcers, and Crohn's syndrome. When our digestive system is not functioning properly, it affects everything else in our body. But what we eat is essential for our health: how our body digests our food is imperative for the regeneration of the cells throughout our body. There can also be physical interferences with the nervous system affecting spinal alignment. When we ignore these symptoms, we become more susceptible to complicating our health problems even further, which can lead to all types of cancers and especially colon cancer. As we become conditioned to mask symptoms, we lose sight of the basic reasons of indigestion. When we overindulge in food; consume the wrong types of carbohydrates, proteins, and fats; and drink artificially flavored drinks with copious amounts of sugar and other chemicals, it seems obvious how illness can proliferate. When we listen to the wisdom of our body, it can be as simple as realizing, "I overate at the party last night; I had too many desserts, drank too much alcohol, went to bed late, had a restless sleep, and woke up feeling bloated, congested, and constipated." When we become disconnected from our body's wisdom, we ease our pain with the latest drugs and continue abusing our health, causing more and more complicated conditions that then require more complicated prescriptions and surgery. Everyday healing is not about being perfect but instead about having an inner compass and consciousness regarding our health that responds to our circumstances in a healthy manner.

DIGESTIVE ENERGETIC PARADIGM

Create a quiet, comfortable space with yourself:

1. First begin to ask yourself, what is my body trying to tell me?
2. Have I been eating the wrong foods or overeating?
3. Have I been physically tired and rundown?
4. What do I feel like I am holding on to or suppressing?

Why is my abdomen hurting? I am upset with _____ (use the person's name).

I am upset with _____ because _____ (core issue).

I feel _____ (core emotion) when _____.

What I tend to do when I feel this way is _____ (type of behavior).

How this affects the relationship is _____.

I then begin to feel _____.

As I hold on to these feelings, my body begins to feel _____.

As my body feels _____, I feel _____ about myself.

Instead of having indigestion, constipation, or abdominal pressure, I would like to create _____.

Instead of holding on to these thoughts and feelings, what I would like to create is _____.

If I were creating _____, I would begin to feel _____ about myself.

If I were feeling better about myself, my relationship with _____ could then _____.

I can now imagine my health and my relationship with _____ evolving in healthy ways.

This is an example of how this exercise can be completed.

I do not really know why my stomach is hurting. I can't think of anything that I am upset about. When I think about it now, I realize that I am upset with my boyfriend, Sam. I am upset with him because he does not seem as affectionate and loving as he once was. I feel frustrated when he criticizes everything I do. I then tend to judge him and reject him sexually at bedtime. I am beginning to feel hopeless in our relationship, as we are becoming more critical of each other. I then begin to feel that any relationship I am in will ultimately fail, causing more suffering in my life. As I hold on to these thoughts and feelings, my body hurts, I feel drained, and my abdominal area feels stuck. Everything I eat seems to cause a lot of gas, and I don't feel energetically happy and alive. As I feel all these things, I feel like a failure yet somehow wish things could improve. What I truly would like to create is becoming healthier and feeling better about myself. I now can see that if I was feeling better about myself, I would be less critical and judging of Sam as well. I can see how I have not been communicating in a compassionate, loving way to Sam, and I am now ready to create healthy communication where I am being more responsible for my own frustrations.

What I want to create is a passionate, healthy relationship with Sam where we are both committed to our relationship. I am committed to express myself emotionally and sexually in a loving, tender way that empowers our relationship. Even as I do these exercises, I can see the difference between wishing for something to improve and creating what I desire. I now feel more energetic, more alive, and more connected to the possibility of creating vibrant wellness, body, mind, and spirit. I am excited about a new possibility in this relationship, now that I have allowed myself to look deeply at how I was feeling.

As you begin to explore these exercises, begin to experience how holding on to these feelings affects all your relationships, your life, and your health.

This exercise could have also reflected a relationship regarding yourself.

I am upset with myself because I continue to eat the wrong foods and continue to gain weight. I am upset because I know these are the wrong foods, and I continue to fool myself. I feel frustrated, helpless, and weak because I do not keep my agreements with myself. When I am feeling down, frustrated, and lonely, I tend to crave the wrong foods and eat more to suppress my feelings. As I continue to do this, I feel worse about myself and continue to suffer. I then feel like I am getting even more depressed and just want to take some drug to not feel anything. As I hold on to these feelings, I can see that my health is declining, and the possibility of being in a healthy relationship with anyone else is impossible.

What I would like to create is a healthy relationship with myself, where I am nurturing myself physically, emotionally, and spiritually. I want to become more disciplined with nutritional eating and exercise. I want to feel better about myself by being kinder to myself and let go of making myself wrong for what I have not accomplished in the past. I can see that if I took this one day at a time, I would begin to have more energy, feel more creative in my life, and lose necessary weight. I now am beginning to feel excited about a new possibility regarding my health, my healing, and the possibility of sharing my life with someone else in a powerful, healthy way.

MUSCULOSKELETAL PAIN
(WEIGHT OF THE WORLD, STIFF NECK, INFLEXIBILITY, RIGIDITY, INSTABILITY, LACK OF SUPPORT, SHOULDERING THE BURDEN, RESISTANCE)

EVERY DAY, PEOPLE complain of backaches, knee pain, lower-back pain, neck pain, shoulder pain, and other joint-related problems. There is an endless supply of medications that ease the pain while the conditions of these problems become worse. Eventually as people get older, we are diagnosed with degenerative joint and muscle problems that often require surgery and stronger medication. As we are diagnosed with forms of arthritis, fibromyalgia, carpal tunnel syndrome, and osteoporosis, we often are led to believe that these degenerative joint diseases are a natural process of aging. When we are not listening to the wisdom of the body, it certainly can appear that way, yet all these ailments begin when we are young.

In America we have all been educated from early ages how to take care of our teeth and prevent serious periodontal problems. Yet just the opposite is true for the rest of our body. We all recognize that small cavities can become bigger cavities if not corrected, and we all understand simply masking the pain does not correct the periodontal disease process. When we do not understand the simple aches and pains when we are young, our body has little choice other than developing more serious aches and pains as we become older. Even the so called growing pains that often have been labeled as the cause of a young person's pain are not an accurate description of a young person's developing body.

The simple truth is our body is being used each day and often when we are young; our body is stressed by ongoing falls, vigorous activities, and occasional injuries. Our musculoskeletal body supports us and allows us to be creative and active in our life.

The term *repetitive stress trauma* has been used to describe the nature of many joint conditions, particularly carpal tunnel problems where the median nerve is being trapped between the small muscles, bones, and joints of the wrist. Often people will receive strong drugs to attempt to reduce pain and inflammation, before the recommendation of surgery. What is observed regarding the wrist and termed as a repetitive stress trauma can actually be applied to most ailments in our body. The term speaks for itself. Repetitive means something that is continuously being performed. Stress means that the very nature of the activity is aggravating and wearing down an area of our body. Trauma means that in this case the trauma is not from an accident, but instead something that takes place over a long period of time.

When we begin applying everyday healing in our life, repetitive stress disorders can be prevented and reversed. Even though we are addressing musculoskeletal conditions in this section, repetitive stress disorders can be related to all degenerative diseases including most cancers, heart disease, and diabetes. When we become conscious of our everyday habits and everyday symptoms, small problems never need to become larger. Discover which healthy strategies are not being implemented or are out of balance in your life. Do you have an ongoing stretching routine at home and at work? Do you receive body work in the form of massage, chiropractic, acupuncture, reflexology, Pilates, yoga, kinesiology, and other healthy modalities?

Musculoskeletal Energetic Paradigm

1. First ask yourself, what is my body attempting to tell me?
2. Have I been eating healthy?
3. Have I physically been pushing my body?
4. Did I do any new physical activity that I have not done in a while?
5. Do I feel I am resisting something in my life?

I feel responsible for _____ in my life.

Where I feel I am not being supported in my life is related to _____.

When I feel that I am not being supported, I feel _____ in my body.

When I feel I am not being supported, I tend to _____.

How this affects my health and the relationships I am in is _____.

Where I am having a difficult time with change in my life is related to _____.

Where I feel I am being stubborn in my life is related to _____.

Where in my life do I feel I am being judged? _____

Where in my life I feel I am being critical and judging is _____.

When my muscles feel tight, I also feel inflexible relating to _____.

When I feel inflexible and resistant to change, it affects my health _____.

When I am feeling unsupported and feeling responsible for everything, I would like to create _____.

Rather than feeling judged and also judging others, I would like to create _____.

What I want to create relating to my health and relationships is _____.

Something I know I can start to do immediately is _____.

What I want to create in the relationship with myself is _____.

This is an example of how this exercise can be completed.

I feel responsible for everything in my life. I do not feel supported by anyone in my life. I feel I am on my own. Since I am not feeling supported by anyone, I feel ongoing stress and pressure and tightness in my body. When I feel unsupported, I tend to have moments of working harder and then moments of giving up. This affects my health and relationships in a negative way. I am not feeling as healthy as I used to feel, and I feel there is no room for a healthy, intimate relationship in my life. I feel rigid and stuck as I think about changing the way things are. I can feel my muscles and joints become tighter as I feel inflexible in my life. I know this is affecting my sleep, my energy, and my overall health.

What I would like to create is joy and fun regarding my life. I would like to create honoring myself and feeling good about being responsible in my life. I would like to create the ease of supporting myself and acknowledging each day my strengths and positive virtues. I would like to recreate my relationship with God and feel the divine presence of his love. I would like to create a connectedness with my body and feel resilient and flexible again. I want to create the possibility of a wonderful love affair that could grow into a committed, supportive relationship. I feel I can immediately begin to start stretching, meditating, saying positive affirmations, and receiving healing work on a continuous basis to empower my new commitment to myself.

CHAPTER 30

CHEST AND BREATHING PROBLEMS
(SHORTNESS OF BREATH, ANXIETY, BREATH OF LIFE, FEAR)

WHEN WE HAVE not been breathing healthy for years, it is easy to forget how essential breathing is to our physiological and emotional well-being. One of the first complications children face is asthmatic conditions. From the trauma of childbirth, our body is being stressed and adapting to breathe shallow through our mouth rather than breathing in through our nose and out our mouth. As our breathing becomes more shallow and restricted, it depletes life's oxygen replenishing every cell, every muscle tissue, and every organ in our body, as well as letting go of carbon dioxide, one of our body's waste products. In a sense the simple equation should be the more life we breathe in and the more toxicity we breathe out, the healthier our mind and body can function. For most of us, it is just the opposite. We breathe in minimal life and breathe out minimal toxicity, causing an ongoing degenerative process where free radicals proliferate throughout our body. There is a whole exercise regimen related to aerobic activity to ensure the mind and body is balancing its oxygen and carbon dioxide ratio. Yet what about people who cannot do aerobic activity? Their body has no opportunity other than to continue to adapt to the circumstances. When we learn everyday healing, we realize that everyone at every age regardless of illness can begin to create strategies to empower their health. Everyone can learn breathing exercises and simple stretching routines that stimulate nerves, circulation, and cellular regeneration.

DR. MARTY FINKELSTEIN

Anytime someone has an injury, there is a shortening of one's breathing pattern. Anytime we feel afraid, our breath immediately constricts. As we continue to worry on a daily basis, our breathing patterns become more and more shallow. Every thought affects our breathing either in an expansive manner or a contracted manner. The first exercises I show each of my patients are breathing and stretching exercises to awaken the breath of life. I am certain you have noticed that when you vacation to the mountains or the ocean, one of the first things you do is breathe deeply. At that moment you are awakening and reconnecting to the source of your divine power and innate wisdom. Every day if we simply remind ourselves to breathe deeply, we can reconnect to our inner vacation.

Chest and Breathing Energetic Paradigm

1. First ask yourself, what is my body trying to tell me?
2. Have I been eating healthy?
3. Do I feel physically exhausted or fatigued?
4. Can I breathe deeply through my nose and out my mouth effortlessly?

What I feel anxious about in my life is related to _____ (be specific).

My greatest fear at the present time in my life is related to _____.

When I am feeling these emotions, I can feel my breathing and my chest _____.

When I am feeling anxious and begin to worry, I tend to _____.

After I do that, I tend to then feel _____.

How this affects my energy level is _____.

How this affects my work and relationships is _____.

When I enter new relationships with fear and anxiety, I feel _____.

When I feel fear and anxiety, I would like to create _____.

If I were creating _____, I would begin to feel _____.

If I began feeling _____, my energy level would _____.

If I was feeling _____, my breathing would become _____.

As I began to feel less fear and anxiousness, my relationship with others would _____.

If I were not feeling my fears running my life but instead chose to be excited and confident, I would be able to create _____.

This is an example of how this exercise can be completed.

What I feel anxious about in my life is related to money. What I feel the greatest fear about is not having enough money to retire comfortably and enjoy my life. When I feel these emotions, I can feel my chest contract and my breathing become restricted and tight. When I am feeling anxious and fearful, I tend to become depressed and withdrawn. After I am feeling depressed, I tend to feel self-critical and guilty that I am behaving this way. When I am feeling this way, I feel disconnected from my work and my intimate relationships, which begins to cause me to have more fear and worry.

When I am feeling fear and worry, I would like to create the healthy space to allow myself to be all right feeling these thoughts. I believe that if I was feeling okay about my fears, I would begin creating a better feeling about myself and my possible future. I feel that if I simply accepted my fears as part of being human, I would begin to breathe easier and have more energy to create new possibilities in my life where freedom and love could be present. By giving myself the space to breathe deeper, I feel my whole life could transform with a renewed purpose and passion. If I was feeling more passion and excitement, I believe I would feel more peace about the past as well as the future.

CHAPTER 31

HEART
(ATTACKS, ACHES, BROKENNESS, HIGH BLOOD PRESSURE)

HEART DISEASE, HIGH blood pressure, and heart attacks, once thought to be predominantly male problems, have been growing in proportion affecting women and now even more and more children. When there is an absence of everyday healing strategies in our lives, the presence of disease can only continue to grow. According to a new study, there is a definite rise in children with hypertension and high blood pressure. This increase translates into hundreds of thousands of children developing what often becomes a chronic, lifelong condition. According to Rebecca Din-Dzietham of Morehouse School of Medicine, who led the study, "Unless this upward trend in high blood pressure is reversed, we could be facing an explosion of new cardiovascular disease cases in young adults and adults."

Our heart is a vital muscular organ that works all day pumping blood throughout our body attempting to bring oxygen and nutrients to each muscle, tissue, organ, and cell, so that our body can be revitalized and regenerated. When our body is working healthy, our heart, which is regulated by the nervous system, manages to do that job like a symphony conductor orchestrating the balance of life in our body. But as our body is consistently stressed through physical, chemical, and emotional causes, the heart has to work harder to regulate life's blood being transported through arteries, veins, and tiny vessels called capillaries. As internal physiological stress increases in the body, the heart needs to work harder until an inevitable outcome occurs of blood pressure rising beyond normal and healthy standards. As we turn our attention to eating healthy foods that cleanse our body rather than clog it, exercise moderately to ease the daily pressures of life, and learn how to reduce the stress to our nervous system, then the physiological responses in our body begin to recircuit themselves, creating and reestablishing harmony and balance. I have one patient who would always come see me before he was having his health physical for his job. He had to maintain his blood pressure in a specific range to keep his position. He had a history of heart disease, and on a particular visit in the office as we were alleviating his back pain, he observed his blood pressure also was reduced dramatically. Since that time when I see him stroll into the office, I know he is here for his blood pressure adjustment.

Heart Energetic Paradigm

1. First ask yourself, what is my body trying to tell me?
2. Have I been eating healthy?
3. Do I physically feel worn down and stressed?
4. What am I feeling emotionally hurt about?

My heart is hurting because _____ (specific circumstance).

The emotions I am feeling are _____ related to this circumstance.

When I feel these feelings and pain, I tend to _____.

What I tend to tell myself when I am feeling these feelings is_____.

What usually makes me feel better for a little while when I am feeling this way is _____.

How this affects my emotional and physical health is _____.

How this affects the relationships I am in is _____.

In the past when I have felt these emotions, I have decided that _____.

When my heart is hurting, what I would like to create is _____.

When I feel this pain, I would like to _____.

The actions I would like to take are _____ when I am feeling this way.

The conversations I would like to have with myself are _____.

What I would like to create with my physical and emotional health is _____.

What I want to create in the relationships I am in is _____.

This is an example of how this exercise can be completed.

My heart is hurting because I am going through a divorce. I am feeling sad and angry and fearful as I am trying to navigate through all the difficulties relating to this divorce. When I feel these feelings, I tend to become more anxious and fearful. What I tend to tell myself when I am feeling these feelings is a combination of "I can't believe this is happening to me" and "I know somehow everything will work out." When I speak to friends who I can confide in, I tend to feel a little better for a short time. I can tell that my physical and emotional health is on a turbulent roller coaster of stress and tension. My body is feeling pushed, and I am feeling drained and exhausted. The way I am feeling is exacerbating the anger and fear, which is causing more hostile conversations with my spouse. In the past when I felt anger and fearful during times of difficulty, I decided that life is hard and frustrating and that I was unworthy and incapable of being happy and having a wonderful partnership.

When my heart is hurting, I would like to create a deeper sense of peace with myself. When I feel angry and fearful, I would like to create a loving space with myself where it is okay to feel what I was feeling. I would also like to acquire assistance during these times to create a healthier approach to difficult circumstances in my life. I would like to have a clear vision of what I truly want to manifest in my life and have an action plan and strategy to create specific results. I would like to feel good about myself and hear a compassionate voice inside me that inspires and appreciates me. I definitely want to create becoming healthier physically and emotionally, and feel connected to my inner wisdom and spiritual power. What I want to create with my spouse at this time is a healing and healthy divorce where healthy communication can occur and where we are partners in raising our children. I know that if I were manifesting that, I would feel better about myself and truly feel as if I was healing and evolving as a spiritual being.

Too often we do not know our own blood pressure and assume it is fine. Each of us should learn to evaluate our own blood pressure and understand the basic strategies to have a healthy, functioning heart. The wonderful thing is that knowing our blood pressure is simple and very relevant to our own health.

CHAPTER 32

ALLERGIES
(SENSITIVITY, FRAGILITY, SUSCEPTIBILITY, VULNERABILITY)

ALLERGIES RELATE TO our neurological-emotional-immunological system. Allergies are one of the first conditions that infants and children are prescribed medication for. Initially parents are led to believe that these symptoms are childhood illnesses that they will outgrow, yet just the opposite occurs. When we treat the symptoms without addressing the cause of these problems, our immune system is further impaired with the continuation of medication. The relationship with our neurological physiology and emotions plays a vital role in the development of a healthy immune system. Any spinal misalignments causing pressure on sensitive nerves when we are infants can interfere with the neurological communication of our body. Emotional stress, even if it is subconscious, can affect the inherent strength of our immune system, making us more susceptible to allergies. As we become older, our immune system can become more vulnerable and sensitive, allowing illness to become the norm rather than wellness. Too often we never ask ourselves why we are susceptible to pollen or other allergens when others are not. Throughout the year thousands of people take medication for allergies without ever addressing nutritional, physical, and emotional imbalances. Every day I see patients who have been conditioned to believe that their allergies are normal. We have all been raised with the notion that there even is another season besides summer, fall, winter, and spring. The allergy season! When we begin to apply everyday healing, we can begin to discover our need for medication decreases as our neuroimmunological system strengthens.

Allergy Energetic Paradigm

1. First ask yourself, what is my body trying to tell me?
2. Have I been eating healthy?
3. Have I been resting well and sleeping well?

What I am feeling vulnerable and sensitive about in my life is _____ (be specific).

When I feel vulnerable, I tend to _____.

The feelings I have about myself during these times are _____.

When I have these feelings, I then begin to think _____.

How this affects my overall strength and energy is _____.

How this affects the relationships I am in is _____.

What I would like to create when I am feeling vulnerable and sensitive is _____.

The thoughts and feelings about myself I would like to have are _____.

What I would like to do to empower myself more would be _____.

How I would like to empower the relationships I am in is _____.

This is an example of how this exercise can be completed.

I am feeling very vulnerable and sensitive about my weight. When I am feeling sensitive about being overweight, I tend to avoid social gatherings and people. I do not like how I feel about myself during these times. At times I even feel suicidal even though I know I would not end my life that way. When I am feeling these emotions, I begin to think things are hopeless and that I will never be in a loving relationship. It just seems the more I try to break out of this pattern, the worse things become. When I am feeling these thoughts, I feel drained, tired, and stressed. When I am like this, all my relationships suffer, and I do not even want to be in any intimate relationships. Just the thought of being in a relationship is frightening. I feel much too vulnerable to open myself to an intimate relationship. I have tried in the past, and I always get hurt.

When I am feeling vulnerable and sensitive, I would like to create feeling at peace with myself. I would like to see the good things about myself and qualities about myself that are special. I would like to accept my body type and weight and not be so hard on myself. I would like to accept that I am not perfect and I may eat the wrong foods at times. What I would like to do to empower myself is find a good wellness coach who can specifically guide me with the proper exercise and nutrition and eating strategies. Ideally I would like to feel good about myself so that every relationship I am in can evolve in healthy ways. Amazingly, as I am doing this exercise, I am already feeling better and more excited about my future. I can truly see that if I was nurturing myself, I would feel better about myself. I know I have a lot to give to others, and the more I love myself, the wiser I can be in choosing healthy people to participate with.

CHAPTER 33

FATIGUE AND DIFFICULTY SLEEPING
(TIREDNESS, BOREDOM, LIFELESSNESS, DEPRESSION, RUNNING ON EMPTY, ANXIETY, SLUGGISHNESS, WEAKNESS)

WE ARE BECOMING so addicted to medication that often we need a drug to help us sleep and then a drug to pep us up in the morning to begin the day. Sadly, the pattern of this cycle continues to wear down our immune system and nervous system. The more we treat the symptoms, the weaker and more fatigued our body becomes. When we are tired, we feel uninspired. We tend to push through the day and then collapse in front of the television at night. It becomes easy to think that we are tired because of the long hours of work and the various stresses in our life. It is difficult to observe ourselves objectively when we feel like the victim of our own circumstances.

As our body becomes further weakened, we become more susceptible to disease. Clearly, if we do not sleep well, our body does not have the opportunity to recharge and reestablish its own innate balance. Our body keeps on working hard internally even while we are attempting to rest in our beds. We tend to rationalize our fatigue as "just stress," while we greet the morning with coffee and muffins and drink and eat unhealthy foods throughout the day. Initially our blood sugar levels increase, giving us the illusion of more energy, until like a roller coaster the blood sugar level comes crashing down, leaving us even more tired and weak. We can think of sugar and caffeine like a drug that is stimulating the body to be activated without nurturing the body with the proper nutrients to strengthen the body's energy throughout the day. Even though our body is tired by the end of the day, most people cannot fall asleep because their mind is anxious and cluttered with stressful thoughts. When this pattern continues, even the most outwardly successful people become depressed. Depression medication has become a lifestyle for so many people claiming it as a disease rather than observing the core physical, emotional, and spiritual imbalances that can be manifesting.

Dr. Marty Finkelstein

Fatigue and Difficulty Sleeping Energetic Paradigm

1. First ask yourself, what have I been feeling about my life?
2. What have I been eating?
3. What have I been doing creatively in my life?

What I feel tired about in my life is _____ (circumstance).

When I don't sleep well, my energy level tends to _____.

When I feel tired and fatigued, I usually like to eat _____ (foods).

When I cannot sleep well at night, I tend to _____ (activity).

When I feel worn down, this makes me feel _____ (emotion).

When I feel _____, I tend to _____.

When I am feeling tired and _____, it affects the relationships I am in _____ (positively or negatively).

When I am bored, I like do _____ (activity).

How I feel about myself when I am bored and rundown is _____.

What I would like to create or recreate in my life is _____.

What I would like to do to start having more fun in my life is _____.

The changes I would like to create regarding my eating patterns are _____.

What I would like to do to help me sleep better is _____.

Some new healthy commitments I am willing to make with myself are _____.

This is an example of how this exercise can be completed.

What I feel tired about in my life is the same routine each day. When I don't sleep well, my energy level decreases. When I feel tired and fatigued, I usually crave sweets. In the evening it is difficult to fall asleep because of a lot of anxious thoughts. I tend to toss and turn and occasionally get up and watch television until I fall asleep. In the morning I feel worn down, yet I just push myself through the day. I pretend that everything is fine with my coworkers and family members. I tend to keep my feelings to myself, and I know this is not healthy for the relationships I am in. I feel horrible that I am in this situation, but I feel like I am stuck and do not have enough energy to do anything different.

What I would like to create is having more fun in my life. I am going to start writing down goals and find people to assist me in achieving the goals I want to accomplish. I know that if I begin creating healthy strategies for my life again, I will seek out eating healthy foods as well. When I am feeling better about myself, I tend to eat healthier and also have more energy. I can see that there is a repetitive cycle that is easy to fall into where things continue to get worse. I now believe I can change that pattern and truly begin changing my life where more joy and happiness would be present.

CHAPTER 34

DEPRESSION, ANXIETY, AND NERVOUSNESS
(OUT OF BALANCE, MOODINESS, UPTIGHTNESS, SUPPRESSING, DEPRESSION, DISCONNECT, JUST STRESS)

THE MARKET FOR depression medicine has soared over the last ten years. We have seen the symptoms of stress and anxiety increase in all age groups as well as financial groups. Sadly, in most cases instead of people improving, the need for more medication has increased. As we depend on the medication, we become further alienated from ourselves, ultimately becoming more depressed. Our true job of healing is not to numb our feelings but awaken our true self and discover where our woundology resides. Where are we hurting? Where are we feeling disconnected from ourselves? We have become a nation of suppressing and numbing, ignoring, and pretending when it comes to the most miraculous life form on our planet, us. Children now are on numerous medications for anxiety disorders that can be unnecessary when we approach each person individually and explore where the cause of the imbalances may be coming from. Each of us has had feelings of being wounded in our life. We have all been hurt in some way. We have all felt insecure, uncertain, and rejected, and from the earliest of ages, we have felt feelings of not being good enough, smart enough, worthy enough, or attractive enough. Regardless of how much we would want to thwart these feelings, they exist at some time for all of us. At the earliest age, children develop survival adaptations to get through the day.

Hopefully at some point we can give ourselves permission to feel the root core of these feelings and recognize that all of us are here to learn and evolve as spiritual persons capable of discovering conscious lessons of life that assist us in truly fulfilling our life's work, purpose, and dreams. Sadly, the age group with the highest rate of suicide is teenagers. They feel the confusions and pressures of life and do not have a healthy atmosphere to communicate about their thoughts and feelings.

Dr. Marty Finkelstein

Depression, Anxiety, and Nervousness Energetic Paradigm

1. First ask yourself, have I been taking care of myself?
2. How have I been eating? How have I been thinking about food?
3. Where in my life do I feel shutdown? Where do I feel creative?

At the youngest age, I remember being anxious about _____ (circumstance).

I remember that when I was anxious regarding _____, I would feel_____ (emotion).

At the earliest age, I began to believe that I wasn't _____ enough.

How I tried to compensate for those feelings was by _____.

When I feel depressed, I tend to _____ (activity).

After that I then feel _____.

My greatest fear if I tried to change this pattern of anxiety would be _____.

What I would like to do but never seem to have the time for is _____.

What I would like to learn that I have not had the time for is _____.

What I usually feel when I do not participate in those areas is _____.

What I want to start doing differently in my life is_____.

What I am going to do to begin feeling better about myself is _____.

I can see that if I managed my time better and kept my agreements with myself, I would begin to feel _____.

The people in my life who I want to share my feelings and thoughts with are _____.

I can imagine that if I share my feelings in a powerful way, these relationships will _____.

This is an example of how this exercise can be completed.

I can remember at the earliest age feeling anxious around family members. I can remember feeling awkward and shy. I can remember feeling at an early age just not being good enough or smart enough. As a coping adaptation, I believe I became rebellious and desired to create my own journey, my own path. When I feel depressed, I tend to withdraw, distancing myself from others. I usually feel worse after that because I feel I am damaging healthy relationships I am in. My greatest fear is failing or feeling rejected. If I had more time and didn't feel so tired, I would love to travel more. I would love to take dance classes, guitar classes, and computer classes, even begin to learn another language. When I desire to do these things but do not take action, I begin to feel hopeless and lost.

What I want to start doing in my life is organizing my time more and keeping agreements to myself. I know if I just begin with one thing at a time, I will start feeling better about myself. I can see that if I write down my goals with specific action steps, I will be creating what I say I truly desire in my life. I want to be honest with the friends in my life and my romantic partner so that they can be a healthy support for my healthy journey. I can imagine that these relationships will also grow deeper and become authentic friendships. I can imagine my partner appreciating my desire to open my heart and my willingness to share my feelings. I can see how that would empower the intimacy of our relationship.

CHAPTER 35

RECONNECTING WITH OUR UNIQUE WISDOM

As YOU DO the healing energy exercises, you will discover how judging and critical we can sometimes be of ourselves. These exercises allow us to observe the inner dialogue that is a continuous loop that disconnects us from our powerful self. The first part of each exercise portrays our survival self that has learned set patterns of behaviors that have existed for many years. When we look at how we respond to situations, the answers come quick because the information is already in our old subconscious brain. When we feel this, we then respond like this, and then we feel this, and then we tend to do this, until we are exhausted, depressed, and sick. Any time we are feeling any stress in our lives, we can explore the true conversation that is subconsciously affecting our lives. In the second part of the exercise, we now can make the transition from subconscious behavior to conscious behavior and make clear, healthy choices that can create healing and new possibilities in all aspects of our lives. The answers to these questions do not come forth as fast or as easy, because these answers have to be created. They are not in the storage box of our brain. We at this moment have an opportunity of inventing powerful changes in our life.

As we begin to become healthier, it is important that we reconnect with our unique qualities that sometimes remain hidden from us. Each of us has unique gifts, though sometimes they are waiting to be discovered or rediscovered.

When we bring our uniqueness to circumstances and situations, amazing possibilities can occur that we cannot see at the present moment.

When we are being in our unique power, we are also being in our true passion.

I met Joe while I was dining at a restaurant. While I was eating my dinner, a jazz trio played sexy, sweet music. When my meal was over, I went over to them and shared how wonderful their music sounded. After a few exchanges, they asked what type of work I did. I told them I was a chiropractor. That was when Joe, who was the drummer, said, "I need to come see you." It turned out he had been in an accident where both hands had accidentally gone through a glass door pane, and he had lost nerve sensation to his wrist, hands, and fingers. Not a good thing for anyone, especially a jazz drummer. Well, sure enough, Joe called the next week and began receiving treatment in the office. It was at that time that I learned Joe was also a computer expert and a genius in the gaming industry. Healing on many levels began to occur for Joe. Physically he began to renew his connection with his body. The metaphor of a finely tuned instrument resonated with Joe as he began to feel his energy level improve physically and emotionally. After a few months of treatment, Joe began to feel sensation in his hands. Our relationship grew beyond the typical doctor-patient relationship, and we both shared many stories with each other each time Joe came for a treatment.

One day Joe came in and said he had lost his teaching position and was struggling financially. He mentioned that he had some interviews lined up in the computer industry, yet he said he was even thinking of taking a normal job just to make some money to get through these hard times. It was clear Joe was out of balance with his unique power and innate wisdom. Fear, worry, and anxiety were dominating his thoughts and feelings, while weakening his body. As he lay on the table, I began to have Joe reconnect with his unique power. I had him imagine his body and energy like a fine-tuned instrument as the rhythms of jazz pulsated through his spirit. While I gently worked his muscles and touched nerve pressure points, I asked Joe to imagine he was interviewing for the best job possible. I had Joe begin to visualize sharing his computer skills and expertise in the computer industry. But most important, I had Joe sharing this information from his musician spirit and jazz soul. A thousand computer experts can all talk about computers, but what separated Joe from them was his unique genius. I asked Joe to visualize from both hemispheres of his brain—his left logical brain and his right creative brain. Muscles began to relax, energy began to flow, and a feeling of balance and vitality became present. Joe felt very excited after his treatment.

Not only did Joe end up getting the job, but in a short time Joe was one of the main leaders in the gaming industry. Typically, our own unique genius is simply being courageous in who we truly are. When we try to be like others and sound like others and fit in rather than being our unique self, nothing distinguishes us from everyone else. As we heal we reconnect to our own true inner power and discover possibilities for our life that were unimagined or unobtainable before.

What are some of your creative, unique qualities?

Review

Well, you have gone through A–Z and More. Congratulations! Now it is essential to apply this in your life.

Recommendations

1. Every day read one section of A–Z beginning with the letter A: Attitude/Action. Discover how you can integrate this information into your life. After completing all the letters over the next twenty-six days, simply begin again. Also, if you are being faced with any challenge in your life, open the book to any random page and see how that message may assist you through whatever difficulties you may be facing.
2. Take the time to stretch and breathe every day.
3. Be mindful of any stress you are feeling.
4. Think of three things you appreciate about yourself.
5. Share appreciations with others.
6. Connect with nature.
7. Share your love with the people you love.
8. Be kind and compassionate.
9. Take a wow walk.
10. Eat nutritious, healthy food.
11. Feel connected to your spiritual power.
12. Begin to create a journal, and at least once a week, begin to do the emotional exercises. As you begin the process of becoming healthier, you will discover that doing these exercises become easier for you. As you allow yourself to feel what you feel, the process of healing becomes natural.

13. Remember, each of us can become healthier, feeling more energy and vitality in our lives, if we are willing to make changes in our lives. There is no shortcut, but there are simple guidelines that, if followed, can create predictable, positive results in our life.

I can imagine a time when all health care professionals work together to help others navigate this journey of wellness and healing. Our real health insurance is available to everyone.

About Dr. Marty Finkelstein

Dr. Finkelstein has been a holistic chiropractor since 1980 specializing in physical, nutritional, and emotional healing in Decatur, Georgia. He is the creator of the workshop "Have the Relationships You Desire," and he has been the host of television, radio, and Internet shows, educating and inspiring others to greater health. He has been the chiropractic representative for Flying Doctors of America, traveling to others countries and providing service alongside dentists and medical doctors.

He is the author of several books, including:

A Life of Wellness
The Seven Gifts
Divorce: An Uncommon Love Story
If Relationships Were Like Sports, Men Would at Least Know the Score
8 Lessons for Life on Hole 1
A Healing Journey—a Collection of Songs

These books can be ordered online through Amazon or by contacting Dr. Marty Finkelstein.

Dr. Marty Finkelstein can be reached for individual healing coaching, workshops, or motivational talks to empower our lives.

www.mydecaturchiropractor.com
http://drmartyswellnessexperience.wordpress.com
drmarty3@yahoo.com